At Walking Pace

A short journey through the wonder of walking

Nyla Naseer

Published by Temblem Publishing

Copyright © 2020 Nyla Naseer

ISBN: 978-1-8382422-2-0

Acknowledgements

At Walking Pace is a book built on many years of walking and reflection undertaken by me at different points in my life. I wish to acknowledge the role of the many friends who have accompanied me on the journey. This includes fellow walking group members, walk leaders, co-workers and other people who have just liked to walk.

At Walking Pace was written during the Covid-19 pandemic, I am appreciative of the fact that, had it not been for the pandemic, I would not have been encouraged to galvanise my passion for walking into a book.

I wish to thank fellow writers in Birmingham, England for their support and guidance.

CONTENTS

Introduction

This is a book about walking. That's right, walking. If you think you know everything you need to know about walking, and that comprises the one foot in front of the other motion you use to get about going from one room to the next, think again. Walking is a humble and un-heralded phenomenon that is only now starting to be fully understood as useful to many aspects of our lives, way beyond the physical benefits of getting moving. Indeed the more you learn about it, the more remarkable the simple act of walking becomes.

Walking has been around forever (in human existence terms) and has had its moments in history; however the breadth and depth of its benefits to all of us have been little researched and written about. I want to change that by presenting a concisely comprehensive overview of how you can benefit from walking right now and why it is time for a walking renaissance. This is a gentle walk though the research and experiences that celebrate the role of walking, not in a chest-thumping way but in a human-scale and practical way that I hope you can relate to.

Walking is the most natural means of getting around under your own steam and the only sustained dynamic exercise that it is possible for nearly all of us to participate in (even if we go slowly at first). No special skills or equipment are required and you can do it anywhere. Walking is flexible enough to be accommodated into occupational and domestic routines, as well as for leisure or specific fitness training. It is self-regulated in intensity, duration and frequency, and, as a low-impact activity, is inherently safe. Unlike so much physical activity, there is little, if any, decline in walking potential in middle or older age. It is a year-round, readily repeatable, self-reinforcing, habit-forming activity and the main option for increasing physical activity in sedentary populations.

I want to enlighten you to the ways that walking can enhance your life, whether you want to start walking in earnest for health or wellbeing reasons, or because you are curious about just how walking can make an impact on your life. Using a combination of research study information, observation and my own experience I have summarised the ways that you can use walking in your life. I've also looked into the extra elements that can enhance your experience of walking and the benefits that it brings you; for example, does playing music whilst you walk make a difference, or should you try some problem-solving whilst you are on the move?

Introduction

Just to let you know, I'm not typically someone easily lured by the prospect of cure-alls and quick fixes. Indeed, it is partly as a response to my concern with the way that people are piling into faddish lifestyle changes including dietary regimes and overly-stringent physical training that I am sharing my take on a natural, easy to implement, low-drama and low-risk activity that, in my view, can be a metaphor for a new way of living. Instead of piling your hope into the next influencer-backed gadget or concoction, why not trust your own instincts and go for a walk? There has never been a more appropriate time in history to do this.

My personal story is deeply relevant to my curiosity about and interest in walking. I didn't much think about it at the time but walking has carried me through some pretty grim periods of my life, as well as being at the heart of the best times. It is only when I've looked back and considered the impact of walking in my life that I've realised just how important this constant 'friend' has been. The interesting thing has been that nothing has prompted me to open the door and walk; it has been an innate sense that walking is a solution and a joy that has driven me to walk. Talking to other people, both regular walkers and those who would not call themselves walkers, uncovers that the decision to 'go for a walk' at key times, whether to cool down or to share news or simply to stretch one's legs, is universal and across cultures.

This primal instinct to walk is something that informs our actions at a very subconscious level and that we need to harness and use to its full potential.

My Walking Story

I am a lifelong walker. An early first memory of mine is of a visit to relatives in Germany, where I, as a two year old, embarked on a countryside outing. Possibly a little overwhelmed by the strangeness and excitement of being in a new place, I must have jumped at the chance of going on a bit of a trip outside the city. I recall being on a steep hill (in reality probably a slope) and striding out on my small legs in front of the other people. Noticing that they had dropped behind, I proclaimed in terribly precocious language "come on everybody, let's persevere" The little girl that I was had already discovered that:

- Walking was something that was good;

- Walking encouraged me (and the people around me) to keep going;

- No-one was going to get in front of me on a walk if I could help it!

In common with other children I loved walking. All that stomping through leaves and sploshing though puddles: it was nectar to the soul. Walking seemed the stage for all the little dramas that played out in my early years.

Later, when I was a teenager and young carer, when things got tough I just put on my shoes and walked, for what seemed like hours sometimes, my mind gently letting go of issues and settling into a calm state in time with my footsteps. At that time, as I noted, I did not even think of walking as being a leisure activity: I just innately knew that it was something that would make me feel better about life. In addition it didn't cost anything, a big consideration at the time. Nowadays, with safety considerations, people are reluctant to venture out, especially on their own, but this was at a time when people generally had less of a thing about being out and about and walking made me more confident about handling the stresses of life independently. Navigating different streets successfully was an achievement that was not only practically useful but a metaphor for decision making in general.

I may not have realised it at the time but perhaps because my mother could not walk as a result of her severe Rheumatoid Arthritis, I valued walking as something precious and noticed its importance more than my peers. The frustration of not being able to walk was something I vicariously absorbed and this must have spurred me on to be even more determined to make journeys on my own two feet. To be honest, I also had no choice: as we had no car it was the bus or 'Shanks's pony'. But even without a car, I still felt I had more freedom to roam and explore than other people – relying on walking made me learn to explore.

It was during my university years and my early years at work that I discovered the joys of walking in the countryside. Mixing walking with nature, I had finally found my spiritual home in terms of the whole walking vibe! I discovered a community of people with a shared interest in donning outdoor gear and tramping around, sometimes up hills and sometimes across muddy fields but with the express intention of spending the day walking. I was fortunate in that my arrival on the walking scene coincided with the advent of special initiatives to welcome young people into walking because the average age of hikers in the UK at that time had crept up as the original rambling community carried on walking but new people were not taking up the interest in terms of leisure. Fortunately for me, my local area had a brand new 'twenties and thirties group' that I could join. Though the walking world was overwhelmingly white, I felt immediately culturally part of something that was the real 'me'. Indeed, being part of the walking fraternity meant that I felt a new level of confidence and, facilitated by the sprightly pace of the walks, I discovered the raconteur in me!

With the advantage of a relatively captive audience for my anecdotes and observations on the world I uncovered the role of walking in promoting communication: from the deep and meaningful to the frivolous and banterful. No doubt I bored or irritated quite a few of my walking companions along the route to this enlightenment with my opinions about what was going on in the world, light-hearted musings and deep discussions.

Embracing the amazing efficacy of walking, I started to work it into my daily routine. At work, I'd make excuses in my mind to walk and made walking the punctuation for my day. So, if there was a meeting to attend and it was relatively local, I'd forget the car and walk there instead. With a little planning this was almost always just as quick as driving, finding somewhere to park and all the pfaffing around that goes with using a car for short work journeys. Arriving at these meetings provided an opportunity to share bits of observation I had made en route, which proved to be a good ice-breaker at times. Walking gave me a uniqueness that marked me out as an individual rather than a corporate clone. It was not just personality that walking ascribed to me either: I discovered that I walking refreshed my mind and out of nowhere I could pull ideas and potentially useful information. In fact, the more walking I did, the more benefits seem to flow. This was all before even considering the health benefits; okay I felt good, healthy and strong but when you are young I think you take this for granted most of the time.

Walking comes in different formats: from the stroll to the challenging hill hike. I found that the type of walking I did resulted in different gains, so the gentle stroll was excellent for letting my mind wander and the physically demanding hikes honed a quality that I am particularly proud of and interested in: resilience. Once you are familiar with the feeling that you have reached the summit of a 'mountain', or have completed a particular walk with less effort than before, you really feel that sense of toughness that can be translated into different environments. There are arguably more issues that can challenge us nowadays: from the precarious nature of employment to the hurtful nature of social media. Life can be particularly tough for young people, many of whom, naturally, feel under pressure. This has led to the coining of the phrase (unfairly in my view) 'the snowflake generation' indicating a fragility and inability to cope with the slightest setback in life. Yet, with the 'micro-challenges' of normal life being replaced by the ease of technology, we become progressively less able to become more resilient. Since modern life requires a great deal of resilience and there are diminishing opportunities to acquire it without, I consider walking to be an important resilience-fuelling weapon.

My interest in walking as contributing to solutions for almost all of life's problems has come in the last few years. As the routine of everyday became, in some ways, much easier thanks to technology and as we have become ever more hooked on the ubiquitous social media and online leisure pursuits, so there has been a corresponding decrease in activity for most people, accompanied by new problems like rocketing obesity, anxiety, falling productivity and security. The level of anxiety around us all increased and turning to Google for answers just exposed us to more and more faddish advice, or sucked us into the trap of becoming reliant on unhealthy activities. There surely needed to be something out there for people who did not want to stare at a screen all day, something simple and not dependent upon gadgets, or (in an age where it is becoming hard to find and distinguish the real friends from the hangers-on), dependent on anyone else? Moreover, an activity that anyone could do, whatever size or age and without fear of being judged. Something that was progressive, so that you could do more as your enthusiasm and ability improved?

Cue my renewed evangelism about walking. As an antidote to sitting in front of screens, and to tone down all that stress that life today seems infused with a slug of old-school Enid Blyton style adventure, walking seemed, in my mind to fill a void. I started thinking about walking as a service that crossed over so many different areas of life: physical health, mental health, creativity, performance. The more I thought about it, the more convinced I became. As I continued to walk with different groups of people: corporate workers, leisure walkers, people wanting to improve their lifestyle and so on, I learnt and refined my knowledge and thinking about walking as a service. My background in academia enabled me to research walking and confirm or refute my beliefs about the power of the walk. Walking even fitted the bill when it came to my egalitarian philosophy of life: as a great leveller walking was fair and equitable. We could all walk together.

To add to my academic qualifications, I did a Diploma in Personal Training to back up my firm belief that for many people gym sessions don't suit. There needed to be a more user-friendly way to improve fitness that did not depend on image and an unrealistic zeal. I saw the missing link as walking. I started spreading the message about walking and encouraging organisations to think about walking as a way to boost health and productivity.

Then Covid-19 happened. Almost overnight people were restricted in what they could do and not do. Suddenly, people had their personal freedom severely curtailed, not because of war but because of a virus. Lockdown was reality.

For some time, people globally could not participate in social activities outside their own household, apart from almost exclusively online. When restrictions started to loosen (just a bit) in the UK, one of the first things that people were allowed to do was go out for limited exercise. Many people chose to do a daily walk. I remember the other-worldly experience of walking down the street where cars had not moved for weeks, wondering how best to acknowledge the few other people who had ventured out: should I say hi or not? Ultimately, I chose to look empathetically towards them, hoping this conveyed a message that we were 'in this together'.

Then, slowly, people were allowed more contact in progressively larger groups. The unique feature about this progressive loosening on socialising — it had to be in the outdoors. Walking was basically the only exercise everyone could do socially. The number of people walking suddenly rocketed. Out of nowhere people started to flock to local parks and nature reserves. Folk who had never been to the countryside suddenly experienced just how great it was to be walking in the open air. Former treadmill users could compare the experience of walking in nature to walking on a conveyor, people sick of talking on Zoom met up and walked. People working from home popped out for a daily stroll or speed-walk. It was a once in a lifetime opportunity to kick-start the walking movement. Walking became an unexpected superstar of the Covid-19 disaster.

As a result, now is the right time to let people know just how effective walking is. The upsurge in walking is brilliant and for this to become the 'new normal' needs to be underpinned by more than just the lack of any choice. This is the time for a walking revolution!

The next section of the book takes you on a journey through importance of walking as a primal skill and a key stage of our human development. I then go on to look at how walking the history of walking and its importance to culture. Following this I'll be showing you just how useful walking is in terms of physical and psychological health and how it promotes creativity and helps with problem-solving. Furthermore, walking has taken its place as a way to challenge us, both literally and metaphorically.

Walking can and should be integrated much more into everyday life: whether this be at work, as a means of transport or as a leisure or health pursuit. This book enables people to understand the facts about walking and take the first steps towards a walking lifestyle.

At Walking Pace

Walking Back Through Time

Walking is pretty old school. In fact, it is so old school that it is ancient.

Our prehistoric ancestors, it has now been discovered, walked from the offset. Bypassing the 'on all fours' posture of other primates: they walked on two limbs. This feature, along with our relatively massive brains and our ability to make tools is what sets us apart from other animals. The Australopithecus skeleton of 'Lucy', our 3.2 million year old ancestor, with its broad pelvis and thigh bones that angled in towards the knees, clearly showed that she walked about. It seems that bipedalism predates the use of tools and could actually date way, way, back in time to the earliest hominids more than seven million years ago. The 4.4 million year old Ardipithecus ramidus showed extensive evidence of bipedalism (in other words, walking) whilst a six million year old hominid was discovered in 2000 with bipedal thigh bones. (Prang, 2019)

Walking on two feet rather than four requires a radically different physiology. In particular, to propel an animal walking on four legs, the centre of mass must be well forward of the hind limbs in order to give it the propulsion forward which results from forcing the rear limbs against the ground and forward. When we (humans) walk, the centre of gravity is above the supporting leg, so our legs have become longer to drive more force into the ground for propulsion and the pelvis is broader and flatter in order to let us walk with a swinging movement without rocking from side to side. This is what sets us apart from the primates that also walk on two feet, like chimpanzees.

Quite why our ancestors became walkers is not known. Theories have suggested everything from the need for division of labour so that males went out and gathered food, whilst females looked after young early humans; to a response to climate change (Lovejoy, 1988). I can't speak for the domestic arrangements of early man and woman but the idea that food could be gathered by hand (by male and females alike without any other evidence to the contrary) is certainly a plausible reason for walking upright. It is also possible that when early climate change caused a change in environment from forests to grasslands, walking on two feet became a much more energy efficient way of crossing these wide open spaces, compared with moving on all fours. Walking on two legs meant that hands were free to carry things and shoulders, backs and heads could be used to transport bigger objects; humans could now look around, explore and move their homes and communities. This mobility opened up the prospect of travelling to different places and becoming true masters of the space around them.

Walking on two limbs saves about 25-35 percent of the calories that you would need to spend if you were on four (Sockol et al., 2007). This means that more energy was available to feed the brain, which requires an incredible 25 percent of daily calorie needs. The downside is that it is a lot less safe to walk on two legs if you need to be ready to flee from predators; lucky for us then that we are the top predator on the planet. It is easy to see the pay-off in terms of intellect when we went two-legged.

With bigger brains and with eyes that looked straight ahead, bipedalism also made the simultaneous act of walking and talking easier for early hominids. Prehistoric people definitely told stories as they walked in groups, just as we do now. Whilst walking was a necessity, wouldn't early person also have had some occasions when he or she could spend time walking and observing life around them as a leisure activity? I like to think of our ancient relatives enjoying strolling through the forests and marvelling at the views as they got to the summit of a hill, passing on news from their journeys and complaining about life, just as we do now.

So, walking is something that we were born to do. It is in our DNA. Walking is instinctive; anyone who watches a baby's determined efforts to take its first steps will understand just how driven we are to walk. The system for generating rhythmic, alternating activity of the lower limbs for stepping is something you see in the first few weeks of a baby's life (Yang et al., 1998). Once the infant can support itself it rapidly moves toward the one foot in front of the other, heel-planting way of walking that we use through adult life.

We walk based on patterns. It is suggested that innate pattern generators in the spinal cord produce the impulse to step for babies and also generate the basic walking rhythm in adults. As we grow, neural circuits kick in and guide us in the balance and weight distribution we need to adopt to walk. So, the movements we need to walk are programmed into us. Our ancient ancestors would have had the same instinct to walk, an instinct driven by the absolute necessity to range over the land, finding food and protecting themselves from harm.

It is not just the autonomic action of walking that is programmed into our brains: we also instinctively work out where we are going. We have a 'sixth sense' related to the journeys we take. This is hard to see in the world we live in today, where we walk along pre-planned routes (roads); we don't even have to use maps anymore since the advent of satnav. But, hidden in our brains is our own basic satnav system that helps us to work out where to go.

As our ancestors wandered they may also have been innately using a system of walking that mirrors the main way that animals such as honeybees, monkeys and sharks move when looking for food — you may have seen the maps of the wandering paths bees take when foraging for food. Very occasionally, some of the wandering goes out to distant locations, so that there is less 'oversampling' of new food patches. This style of wandering doesn't need much memory or high levels of awareness and, it seems that it works at a subconscious level for living things as a whole. In fact, people in hunter-gatherer societies today (not many of them left to be honest) adopt this 'Levy' walk style: a type of random walk where groups of short step lengths are interspersed with longer movements. This style of walk minimises wasting energy on 'oversampling' a given patch of land and take people to new food patches in the most efficient way and with the minimum of memory and without needing lots of brain-power (Raichlen et al., 2013).

The point I am making with this history lesson is that we evolved specifically to walk in the most creative, useful and effective way possible. Walking is what our bodies were designed to do and, as time has gone on, we have used it in all environments, from the desert to the jungle. This would not be the case if walking was not intrinsically the best way for us to get about.

Let's move on from prehistory to much closer to today: to the age of modern man (Homo sapiens), in other words, someone living in a society that you will have heard of from your history lessons, or from a documentary on TV. People have been walking, primarily as the main form of transport and, more recently, walking by choice (going for walks, hikes, strolling around town etc) and they have been walking everywhere. As people's movement went from wandering to conquering, walking has been a key feature in the growth of major civilisations: in ancient Egypt and Mesopotamia pilgrims and servants made use of roads to travel, predominantly on foot. It is with the rise of the Roman Empire however that walking became a truly formalised civilisation builder. Roads were the skeleton of Roman domination, enabling them to impose order on other places by providing, in the case of the best-constructed roads, an almost perfect fast walking environment. In Europe, pilgrimages were an important part of medieval life; indeed many of these old pilgrim trails still attract large groups of walkers and believers to this day (Caminos). Pilgrimages appear in the itinerary of all the major faiths, from the

Catholic pilgrimage to Lourdes to the Hajj of Islam. These walks — long distance hiking trails in today's language — led to codes of etiquette and fashion that create a bond between the walkers. There are also codes of behaviour that exist between general walkers that echo respect and common sense and defy the impersonal and detached demeanour we adopt in cities. So, fellow walkers will say hello, or give way to others or hold gates open (on the whole) when encountered on a walking trail.

When it comes to thinking, what better catalyst than walking? Monks in the Middle Ages certainly did their fair share of tramping about whilst ruminating. The Dominican, Saint Thomas Aquinas, for example, is estimated to have walked more than 9000 miles in his intellectual meanderings across Europe in the thirteenth century. St Francis of Assisi also piously walked across Europe, attracting many to his group of joyful paupers, demonstrating that even in the thirteenth century materialism was seen as a burden for some who found more happiness in a simpler way of life, underpinned by walking of course. The seminal fourteenth century work by Geoffrey Chaucer: The Canterbury Tales, is set on a journey (okay they may have been riding horses as well as walking) of group of pilgrims as they travel together from London to Canterbury to visit the shrine of Saint Thomas

Becket at Canterbury Cathedral. The insight the medieval journeys of the rowdy and over-sharing travellers, give into the sophisticated minds and lives of people at the time, is, in my mind, made possible by the place of walking in their contemporary lives. Walking gives a timeline to their story-telling. It seems that in medieval England, as people walked, they experienced a sense of wellbeing and the need to communicate: just as we do now.

Historically, walking has proved to be an excellent catalyst for philosophical thinking. I'll go into much more detail about walking and the mind later on, but you can easily see how, when the potential for other distractions so much more limited in the past, both thinking and walking were a bigger deal. In fact, walking may be viewed as the ultimate mind expanding pastime, valued by thinkers of the past for its simplicity and the existential quality that it holds. This was something very attractive to philosophers. By entering a state that we would nowadays call 'mindfulness', or even by enduring a level of hardship caused by fatigue or hunger, great thinkers were able to lose their identity and, unencumbered by concerns of everyday life, they were able to develop their thinking and concepts. Some wandered slowly, others more quickly, but walking oiled the cogs of their minds. I feel strongly that walking and thinking innately go hand in hand. How many times have you gone for a walk around the block to think things over? Probably not as many as the old philosophers but if you have you are following the great traditions of celebrated writers and questioners.

Many creative writers are known to be avid walkers. Charles Dickens, Virginia Woolf and Henry David Thoreau all liked to take walks as part of the creative process. Perhaps the most celebrated walker-writer was William Wordsworth, who always seemed to be ambling down country lanes, hiking up mountains or wandering 'lonely as a cloud'. Other authors centre their stories on the idea of walking: just think of the journeys in JRR Tolkien's 'Lord of the Rings' for example. Walking, for many writers, past and present, is a way to access the inner-self and to leave the outside world behind. Once walking, it feels like you can really open up your imagination and access parts of your subconscious. This may also explain why people on pilgrimages can feel closer to God, or feel that they see visions.

Philosophers such as Nietzsche, Rousseau, Kant and Thoreau all spent a great deal of time walking. Indeed Thoreau famously said: 'Me thinks that the moment my legs begin to move, my thoughts begin to flow.' Nietzsche, famous for uncompromising criticisms of traditional European morality and religion, reportedly spent up to eight hours a day walking, alone, with a notepad in which he jotted down his thoughts and constructed the contents of his books, including, appropriately 'The Wanderer and his Shadow'. He saw his walking route as his office and applied himself to his work of writing with a discipline that he saw reinforced by the act of walking and reflected in his brisk walking style. For Nietzche, walking was an integral part of his work as a thinker and writer.

'All truly great thoughts are conceived by walking.'— Friedrich Nietzsche

The eighteenth century German philosopher, Immanuel Kant, who concerned himself with the concept of nature, ethics and political philosophy based on the concept of freedom, saw walking as a way of escaping and as a distraction from his work rather than part of the process of thinking. Kant's daily brief walks proved enough to sustain him through the rest of his day, during which he philosophised. He walked, as many of us do today, through a park (a route that came to be known as 'The Philosophers Walk'). Kant walked in a predictable, consistent way that gave him the routine escape from writing that he needed to produce his work.

Rousseau, the great Swiss philosopher and social commentator, also made walking a mainstay of his life and work. At the end of a tumultuous life writing stridently against the thinking of the power-mongers of the time on political philosophy and education, he became much more introspective and turned to walking to inspire his thoughts about his own life and a society by which he felt rejected. Writing his thoughts on playing cards as he walked, he worked on 'Reveries of a Solitary Writer', a series of essays based on ten random walks on the outskirts of Paris in which he explored his feelings about life and society, coupled with observations of the sights he saw along the walk. The use of the walk for self-understanding has never been so brilliantly demonstrated.

Want more examples of walking inspiring thinking? Great, because walking itself has generated plenty of comment from an academic perspective. There is a notion that walking itself is a metaphor for social existence: we walk through life. Walking may even by integral to learning in a way that is yet to be fully understood but has a long history. Here is a sprinkling of quotes (available widely) about walking, you've maybe read some of them before; it seems that I'm not alone in considering walking to be transformational:

'Meandering leads to perfection.'— Lao Tzu.

'If you are in a bad mood go for a walk. If you are still in a bad mood go for another walk.'— Hippocrates.

'It is no use walking anywhere to preach unless our walking is our preaching.'— St Francis of Assisi

'Walking is the great adventure, the first meditation, a practice of heartiness and soul primary to humankind. Walking is the exact balance between spirit and humility.'— Gary Snyder.

Of course western philosophers and writers don't have a monopoly on drawing inspiration from walking or extolling its praises. People of other cultures such as those of native North Americans (for example, Cree people) have long established walking ceremonies and traditions that have inspired campaigning walks of today. Dogrib people of north-west Canada have woven walking into the way that they pass on learning to new generations. Maasai people of east Africa and other nomadic cultures see walking as critical to their identity and livelihood.

Walking customs and performances date back centuries and geographically span the world, with walks and processions being used as rites of passage, the most well known of which may be the Aboriginal 'walkabout' a combination of extended survival, knowledge-gathering and self-reflection. Nowadays, these old walking rituals and customs are packaged and offered as experiences for people wanting to step in the footsteps of those who walked before. Although this brings with it issues of 'cultural appropriation' one can understand the draw of the magic and its promise of transformation.

There are so many metaphors that come into play and make sense in terms of walking, learning and transformation; just like our thoughts, walks may go in many different directions or our feet find a rhythm just as we often learn things by adopting a rhythm of information (for example, of numbers, or words) in our minds. When we learn, we go from stationary to moving our knowledge forward: knowledge and movement go together. The process of walking itself can enhance the basic skills we need to learn. So, for example, walking through stimulating environments could influence learning skills and develop skills such as monitoring and remembering. So, in the dense forests of Malaysia, Jahai and Penan people traditionally walked their way through forest debris, through vines and unpredictable environments; walking through these challenges are thought to enhance the perceptive and cognitive abilities of the forest dwellers. Members of the Dogrib tribe of Canada still live in arboreal forest and practice 'pensive observation': think as you watch, watch as you think. Whilst walking they tell stories en route, creating inter-generational knowledge. Walking and stories go hand in hand. The Dogrib feel that only by walking can the ancient stories be properly understood and observations made to bring them to life. The importance of walking to creating cultural memory is established in so many parts of the world that it surely can't be a coincidence? Walking is a vastly overlooked part of cultural memory.

To recap, walking is a skill that was a primary part of our evolution. We did not start moving around on four limbs and then walk upright: humans were designed to walk. Walking enabled our prehistoric ancestors to range over vast areas, to move from places to avoid disasters and to set up home in places that appealed. It allowed them to open up new frontiers both literally and symbolically.

Our brains are wired to walk. Understanding the mechanism through which walking works with our minds is not something that anyone can pinpoint precisely at the moment, although there is an ever expanding volume of research in this area. What can be said though is that walking appears to aid our thinking, as demonstrated by the numerous writers and philosophers who have used walking as part of the creative process. We are not all creative writers or philosophers of course but we all think and use creativity by virtue of the need to develop ideas in the course of our daily lives. The way that we can harness the creative power of walking is explored later in the book.

Many of us instinctively 'go for a walk' to calm down or take some time out to unwind. The potential for walking to help our psychological health and wellbeing is now widely accepted. Walking in green places is even prescribed medically as an alternative to drugs to deal with anxiety and other mental health issues. However, it is not just us 'feeling better' that walking helps: there are real physiological improvements that take place once we start walking. These changes not only help with our physical health and ability to live more healthy lives over the long-term, they also strengthen our psychological wellbeing.

What is unquestionable is that, for the most part, we are walking less than before. Over the course of the past one hundred years people have gone from working in the fields and walking on rough terrain, to working in sedentary occupations and relying on things other than themselves for transport (horses, trains, cars and so on). As we have lost the habit and routine of walking the majority of us don't experience walking in the countryside much at all anymore, or at least we didn't until very recently. Covid-19 changed things, of course and many people who had never considered walking as something to be done other than as a necessity suddenly found it to be their only leisure and exercise option.

Society is changing also. With greater awareness of climate change-indeed with this becoming the most critical issue facing us post-Covid, finding positive alternatives to cars as a means of transport is of urgent importance. Similarly, the crisis in public health means that governments worldwide are urgently looking for solutions to the obesity epidemic. Why: because obesity costs us a lot of money. In the UK alone, the overall cost of obesity to wider society is estimated at £27 billion. The UK-wide NHS costs attributable to overweight and obesity are projected to reach £9.7 billion by 2050, with wider costs to society estimated to reach £49.9 billion per year (UK Government. 2020). Illnesses and diseases from diabetes to arthritis are directly attributable to the impact of being obese. Yet, one of the simplest ways of changing your lifestyle to one that promotes achieving a healthy weight and reducing your likelihood of being unwell, especially over the long-term is, you guessed it, walking! So, there are societal push and pull drivers for making walking a greater element in all of our lives. This is not a book writing out public health or transportation policy but there is plenty of information out there if you want to educate yourself, or indeed input into this fast-moving area. The trend towards walking in terms of creating a better world will continue.

In the next chapter, I'll be looking more closely at the role of walking in improving our physical health and our current lifestyles. I'll also give some practical examples of what we can do to incorporate walking into our everyday lives.

Walking and Physical Health

Firstly, a short lesson in the physiology of walking. Walking is about moving your body from one place to another by moving your legs, one past the other, again and again. It is a repeated cycle of movements. Essentially, the work is done by your legs but the whole body is involved in terms of maintaining your posture and balance during walking. There are two phases to walking: the first is the stance phase where you are getting ready for lift off. This is divided into the heal strike, support and toe-off phases. Then there is the swing phase: this is the leg lift and swing part of walking. There are several different muscle groups involved in walking including your gluteus maximus and quadriceps and, of course, all of the muscles of the foot and ankle. Walking is a complex function that involves more than just your muscular-skeletal system: it also involves your brain. In particular the neural system generates the patterns of rhythmic activity that we need in order to walk; because we have these patterns we don't even think about walking, as the steps are programmed into our brains.

Human walking is sometimes described as a controlled falling because of the way that the body needs to control its mass over its centre of gravity. The amazing thing is that not only do we do this so successfully, but we do so in a way that attempts to limit energy expenditure whether we are walking fast or slowly: you instinctively know how to walk in the most energy efficient way possible.

So, we are fine-tuned to walk. We can walk on and on for very long periods of time. Some regular walkers can walk twenty miles or so a day with no problem; although finding the time to do this might be a bit of a problem. Remember that in the past people walked because there was no alternative, so walking many miles a day was the norm for most people (and still is for large numbers of people around the world. Contrary to the many people who feel that it is second nature to drive as much as you can, you could say that *not* to walk is unnatural.

We are designed to walk, not sit. Yet we now sit more than at any other time in history. We don't just sit when we are tired. We sit all day. We sit for much of our time at work and many of us sit for much of the time at home too, whilst we spend both our work and leisure time on devices. Even when we go out of our homes we sit in cars or on public transport and sit when we get to where we are going. All this sitting is counter to what we are designed to do – walk.

Too much sitting around causes problems for your body; this is true even for people who take some exercise. One of the main impacts of not moving is on blood circulation. Sitting continuously for three hours has been shown to reduce the body's ability to circulate blood flow to our legs, which may increase the likelihood of problems with our arteries. Sitting around weakens muscles and harms our 'core' strength, so that we are less able to adopt a good posture or maintain our activity for so long. Clearly sitting for most of the day on a regular basis is pretty bad for our physical health.

Even more worryingly, having a sedentary lifestyle with lots of sitting is also likely to reduce blood flow to the brain. Maintaining brain blood flow is vital because the brain needs a constant supply of oxygen and nutrients to function and survive. This matters because less blood flowing to your brain is associated with lower cognitive functioning and increased risk of neurodegenerative diseases. Put in lay terms, that means that people who have a sedentary lifestyle can't use their brains as well (to think about things and perform tasks, such as decision-making and planning) and are more likely to develop diseases that involve the brain, including things like dementia or Parkinson's disease. This is concerning and should make uncomfortable reading for all of us. The good news is that the simple act of getting up from your chair every thirty minutes or so and having a walk around prevents the decline in blood flow. Getting up and moving is an effective way to improve circulation (Carter et al., 2018).

What about the other health benefits that walking brings? Well, although we tend to assume that exercise is a well accepted asset to public health, it has only been relatively recently that moderate activity like walking has been considered to be a useful tool in healthcare compared with other measures such as stopping smoking. In the United States the first Surgeon General's report on smoking and health was published in 1964. However, the first Surgeon General's report on physical activity and health was not published until 1996. Since the 1990s however, physical activity like walking has gained acceptance as a way to lower rates of chronic disease. There is now strong evidence that a lack of physical activity increases risk of premature mortality and many chronic diseases, including cardiovascular disease, stroke, high blood pressure, type-two diabetes, osteoporosis, obesity, some cancers, anxiety, and depression.

Lots of anecdotal evidence and studies point to the health benefits of walking but is it really walking that is bringing the benefits in terms of lower incidences of heart disease or diabetes, for example? Or is it that other lifestyle factors such as whether people smoke, drink a lot of alcohol, are obese etc that really count? To pinpoint the real health benefits of walking I trawled through quite a few peer-reviewed studies — that is studies that are accepted as being scientifically valid. What I found was that walking has a demonstrable positive effect on health and it seems that, particularly for people who are overweight, you don't have to do be a power-walker: just substituting sitting for more walking will make a real difference.

A 2017 study by the University of Maastricht for example, found that walking brought a whole host of health benefits for overweight people who walked more and sat less compared to people who spent a lot of time sitting. Insulin sensitivity, a key marker for diabetes, improved as a result of substituting sitting with light walking and the benefits extended into the day after the activity, showing that the improvements have a lasting effect. Similarly, there were marked improvements in 'good' cholesterol', a reduction in 'bad' cholesterol and a lowering of blood pressure after people spent significant periods of the day walking and doing other light activity. Light walking had a definite positive impact on reducing risks that can lead to heart problems (Duvivier, 2020).

As even light walking seems to be effective way of improving one's 'cardiometabolic profile' it is an ideal way to realistically improve the health of the many, many people who just don't want to take more structured exercise. In fact, less than five percent of us do the amount of exercise that we are advised to, therefore overly ambitious plans are often doomed to failure, especially for the people who would most benefit. So, here's an idea to start off with, one that is a lot more feasible than even coaching people on the 'Couch to 5K'— because a lot of people won't make the transition from couch to 5K without something in between and, unless you are going to be doing 5ks very regularly this is not a long-term lifestyle change for people anyway — the more realistic plan of sitting less and replacing the sitting time with walking and other light activities to start a real change of lifestyle. Unfortunately, modern life is leading us to do less and less activity, even light activity like turning lights on and off in our homes or physically going to do some shopping, so some conscious effort is needed to actually walk rather than sit. It can be done.

But is light walking enough? Is our self-interpretation of light walking arduous enough to make a difference? Another study from Spain found that self-selected walking intensity was actually enough to meet official recommendations to qualify as exercise for most people (de Moura et al., 2011). Since even light walking is useful health-wise I feel that self-chosen walking of any speed should be encouraged. However for those people who want to go to the next level, additional motivation could help: walking in groups or with a walking buddy could be a way forward, with professional guidance if there are health factors.

Okay, so not sitting is great but what about people who want to do more than light walking? Is brisker walking noticeably better for your physical health?

At the moderate level, it seems that walking has even greater benefits. Several studies have shown that moderate intensity aerobic activity, such as faster walking, reduces the risk of cardiovascular disease, diabetes and metabolic syndrome in the general population and, in addition, it also has other beneficial physical health impacts.. Walking helps to develop and maintain muscle and it also helps with bone density and balance. Much of the research in this area has been with post-menopausal women, since they are most prone to loss of bone density. Studies show that women who walk as little as a mile a day have higher bone density than women who walk shorter distances. Regular, moderate walking is also effective in slowing the rate of bone loss (Martyn-St James & Carroll, 2008).

Another, often overlooked element of health is balance. Ever had a day when you thought your balance was off for any reason? You will know how frightening a loss of balance can be if you have experienced it; problems with balance can severely limit your life. As you get older balance makes the difference between being sure-footed and confident and potentially having more falls. About 30% of older adults over 65 fall at least once a year. So balance is a serious issue. Yet again, walking can help. Exercise of many types including things like Tai Chi and yoga can help with balance, as can strength training. As well as these activities, walking also assists with balance and has the additional benefits of requiring you to 'read the ground' in terms of terrain, which helps your mind to adjust gait and shift weight and centre of gravity. These imperceptible small challenges train your mind over time to improve balance. In fact, walking programs improve measures of both static (when you are standing still) and dynamic balance. For people of all ages this brings benefits in terms of walking confidence and posture, which is good for general health (Bemben et al., 2006).

There is, of course, one issue that springs to mind whenever we talk about exercise and that is uppermost in people's minds: weight loss and weight control. As a result of our sedentary lifestyles and poor diet we are now, on the whole, heavier than we have ever being historically and with this comes the numerous health problems that I have already referred to. The precursor to being overweight is the 'metabolic syndrome' that causes poor blood sugar control and cardio-vascular problems: issues that walking can assist with. But what about weight loss itself: can walking help you lose weight?

The good news is that walking definitely helps you to lose weight as part of a healthy lifestyle. Looking at walking programmes between four weeks and a year in length, researchers have found that walking results in healthy weight loss and that a longer programme of walking leads to more weight loss than a shorter program. Weight change with walking programmes tends to be consistent, rather than the yoyo weight swings you tend to get with diet programmes alone. As well as helping you to lose weight, walking is important in maintaining weight control. Since walking is cheap, an everyday activity and is generally possible to do in most environments, it is very useful for both individuals and public health planners as a way to keep weight down over the longer-term, with the associated savings to the health service.

We all know that middle-age is associated with weight gain, but it does not have to be so. A long-term (over fifteen years) American study looked at the issue of whether walking could help with long-term weight control. The answer, as you might expect, was yes. Walking led to less weight gain over the period. The greatest benefit was seen for people (in particular women) who were heaviest to start with. For these people, those with the highest walking levels resulted in weight gain of eight kilograms less over fifteen years compared with people who did not walk much (Richardson et al., 2008). The more walking you do, it seems, the more weight lost and kept off: so some walking is certainly better than none, two hours walking is better than one and an hour a day is better than an hour a week. In fact, each extra half an hour a day of walking was associated with an annual reduced weight gain of a pound. Walking seemed to be the driver for this reduced weight gain, over and above other physical activity (Gordon-Larsen et al., 2008). Put simply, you can stop that middle-aged spread by walking, if you start regular walking when you are younger.

Walking also reduces craving for sugary and high calorie snacks. Taking part in a walk of as little as fifteen minutes has been shown to reduce the desire for junk food in both normal weight and overweight people (Hui et al., 2015). Therefore, taking a fairly short, brisk walk, something that can be easily worked into a normal routine, could be a very useful tool in reducing the urge to eat at times when you may be particularly vulnerable to eating junk — such as when you feel stressed or when snack foods are likely to be hard to resist (such as all those celebrations at work). Taking a short, brisk walk might be especially useful if you are a person who finds it difficult to break the habit of snacking at particular times of the day: you could plan to take a short walk at these times to regulate your cravings.

So, what is the best type of walking for losing weight, helping your cardiovascular system, strengthening your muscles and improving your balance? The first important message is that starting to walk, at any level, is better than not walking. Even light walking helps. However, to really kick-start your health improvements, moving your walking to the next level is going to pay dividends.

Making your walking more aerobic, that is lifting exertion into the zone of over 70% of maximal heart rate will develop and sustain even greater physical health and fitness gains. This means increasing walking speed, the time spent walking and other factors to make walking more of a challenge, for example walking uphill. This will also boost your endurance: sustaining your ability to exert yourself over a longer period.

The physical health benefits of walking come in two stages. Firstly the short-term effects of walking on your health (for example the impact on blood-sugar) and secondly cumulative gains over longer term. This is what you should be aiming for if you want to see benefits long-term in terms of weight-control, bringing type-two diabetes under control or improving your cardio-vascular fitness, blood pressure, back pain, improving respiratory fitness and more!

To move up a level means that you have to gear up your walking to a 'brisk-walk'. This means lifting your walking above the threshold of 'comfort' into the aerobic zone. The average middle-aged person should be able to walk three to four miles an hour (a mile should take about twenty minutes), so a brisk walk should be more strenuous than that. It is definitely worth getting into more strenuous walking if you can as it can be as effective as more conventional exercise in terms of health improvements. Regular brisk walkers can have the same reduction in risk for cardiovascular disease as people taking regular vigorous exercise like running (30-40%). So you don't have to take up a sport to help your heart health: the easy, safe and affordable pastime of brisk walking can be just as effective (Williams, 2013).

Brisker walking also pays off in terms of weight loss. In studies with young overweight men, a few months of vigorous walking (walking for 90 minutes on 5 days a week) led to nearly six kilos of fat loss on average, coupled with a gain of lean tissue (Leon et al., 1979). Brisk walkers also improve their blood sugar control which helps with weight loss since the spikes in blood sugar are flatter; this helps to reduce hunger pangs, so that regular brisk walkers may actually eat fewer calories.

Weight loss is now an accepted part of treatment of type-two diabetes; indeed massive controlled weight loss is known to stabilise diabetes to the point where no medication is needed anymore. The improvements in blood sugar control generated by walking mean that it is an excellent activity for people wanting to lose weight safely as part of their strategy for dealing with type-two diabetes: interrupting prolonged sitting with brief bouts of light walking reduces spikes in glucose and insulin for diabetes patients. Since walking is much more likely to become part of most people's lifestyle long-term than other types of exercise, walking seems a very logical addition to assist with diabetes treatment (Dempsey et al., 2016).

To bring the immense potential of walking to life, I want to share with you the story of my friend Philip, a retired ex-academic who was ten stone overweight, had high blood pressure and had suffered from type-two diabetes for over twenty years. Philip was, understandably, quite down about his situation and retirement had made things even worse, since he no longer had the opportunity to pour his energy into his work and felt that his life lacked purpose. The sudden death of his partner was a wake-up call and he decided to change his lifestyle. This was a very brave step since Philip also has Asperger's Syndrome, which makes change extremely challenging. Despite this, by calling on the inner discipline and will to keep going that he had felt when he was in the army as a young man, Philip started to walk on the South Downs near his home. Starting with just a mile, he upped this to three and then six miles a day. Once his new routine had taken hold he started to become a new man. Not only did he progressively lose weight but after six months he no longer needed medication for any of his conditions. In all, he reduced his weight from twenty-three stone to thirteen and (as you might expect) was unrecognisable. In fact, I recall going to meet him at a railway station and walking straight past him. Losing the weight and controlling his diabetes was not easy for Philip and any drastic change is going to need adjusting to over time but Philip is, it is fair to say, looking forward to the next phase of his life as a far healthier person.

One of the main drivers for the surge in walking is the Covid-19 outbreak globally and the allied limitations on other forms of leisure activity and exercise. Naturally, many people are concerned about their immune function, especially since Covid-19 causes the most harm to people in vulnerable groups with impaired immunity: so elderly people and people with pre-existing health conditions are most likely to die and have more complications due to the virus. Younger people and people with better overall health (including stronger immune systems) on the whole are asymptomatic, or have milder symptoms. So, could walking help to boost your immune system and make you more able to deal with illness and, more specifically, viruses such as Covid-19?

The role that exercise plays in immunity may surprise you. An accepted view is that strenuous exercise causes a drop in immunity during and after the exercise, creating an opportunity for viruses to invade. Lots of different aspects of the immune system show adverse change immediately after prolonged, heavy exertion, which has an impact on different areas of the body (e.g. the skin, upper respiratory tract mucosal tissue, lungs, blood and muscle). Many exercise immunologists believe that during this 'open window' of impaired immunity (which may last between three and seventy two hours) viruses and bacteria may gain a foothold, increasing the risk of infection (Kakanis et al., 2010).

If you are a top athlete or you do a great deal of strenuous exercise you may have reason to be concerned. In fact, evidence does back up this model: top athletes are indeed more prone to infections after they train. However, what about the rest of us? Is exercising at a more moderate level, bad or good for our immunity?

It seems that more moderate exercise does *not* compromise immunity and is a way to reinforce strong general health that maintains good immunity. Studies that look at infections consistently see lower rates when people lead active lifestyles. Experiments also show that exercise can enhance immune responses to bacteria and viruses. Naive T-cells which act against new pathogens and are an indicator of an effective immune system, are boosted by an active lifestyle. Furthermore, being active may actually limit the deterioration of our immunity that happens because of age. Exercise like walking can mitigate the actions of 'bad' cells: controlling inflammation and the oxidative stress with aging and obesity (Nehlsen-Cannarella et al., 1991).

Taking all of the points made about walking and physical health and wellbeing into consideration, it is not surprising that some people are 'self-prescribing themselves 10,000 steps a day to improve their wellbeing and walking is also formally being prescribed, together with other activities such as cycling in what is termed 'social prescribing' (*Cycling and Walking 'on Prescription' in the West Midlands*, 2020). This makes sense as structured programmes of walking 10,000 steps a day over a set period of months have been shown to improve both physical health variables such heart and lung health and also psychological wellbeing and a greater commitment to exercise in the longer term (Morgan et al., 2010).

So, walking is good for your physical health and fitness. No surprise: I believe you already suspected that. Let's wrap up this section with a brief overview:

- Any walking is good. You may think that exercise needs to be vigorous and last a long time. Public health guidelines may have reinforced this belief over time leading us all to think that you need to get hot and sweaty to make a difference to your health and fitness. Whilst strenuous exercise can be great for fitness, it is also unrealistic for a lot of people for many different reasons — personal preference being a key one. The good news is that walking instead of sitting brings an enormous boost to your cardiovascular health, blood pressure, cholesterol and your ability to manage your blood sugar more effectively. The more hours a day you spend walking rather than sitting, the more you gain in terms of your health.

- Most people are pretty good at self-selecting their walking speed, although some might need a bit of help. As you walk more you tend to up your walking speed as you get fitter. Walking further helps retain bone density which is especially important for post-menopausal women. Walking also helps with balance as muscles and coordination are improved.

- Walking is a very effective way of losing weight gradually and, especially, maintaining a healthier weight. If you are a regular walker from a younger age you are less likely to put on the 'middle-aged spread' that many people wrongly assume is an inevitable part of growing older. Brisk walking reduces cravings for sugary snacks, which in turn helps to control weight.

- Brisker walking boosts your endurance and can be as effective as running in terms of health gains and weight loss (but you need to keep it up). Brisk walking is also a good way of improving your appetite control so that you are less likely to eat more than you need.

- In contrast to a lot of strenuous exercise, which some people feel compromises immunity to a degree, walking can actually help your immunity, keep your immunity stronger as you grow older and help you to fight off viruses.

These points could motivate you to put on your trainers or walking boots, or just don your comfy shoes and walk around more during the day. The benefit to your physical health will be significant. However, it is not just the benefits to your fitness that people notice: more and more people are acknowledging just how much walking makes them feel good. Walking, it seems, is a natural source of happiness and a mood lifter. In the next chapter I'll be exploring this and highlighting the growing body of evidence behind it.

At Walking Pace

Walking and Feeling Good

In recent years there has been considerable research into the impact of walking on psychological health and wellbeing that I'd like to share with you.

A few years ago, I was part of an experiment at a local university. The research looked at how people's bodies reacted to stress when they walked in green areas like parks, compared to how they reacted when they walked on streets (in this case the streets of a suburb in Birmingham, UK). Data was gathered, not by asking people how they felt, because that might not be the most reliable way of measuring impact, but by taking measurements via a number of devices attached to the body of the walker; in this case me. Fully kitted out, I set off on one of my regular walks, though local parks and a busy shopping street. The results were revealing. When I reviewed the results — a series of maps with red areas indicating stress on the body and green indicating a relaxed response physiologically — I was surprised. My results were all green, even in the urban areas, whereas the maps of other people showed green and red areas. I had also walked a lot further than the others (it was a self-selected walk). It seemed that my long history of walking may have resulted in my body being less stressed in all environments. Of course, there may be other reasons why I responded in this way but I am pretty confident that a lifetime of walking resulted in my body being able to deal with the pressures around me far better at a physiological level, without me even realising this.

Taking my personal example, I walked a route that I knew and loved. The association of walking with places and memories is something deeply embedded within our subconscious. Studies have shown that places can be a source of comfort to people when they are associated with good times or people that we like. Personal connections then, when accessed through the medium of a walk, can bring an enhanced sense of identity and psychological wellbeing. Although we like to think of a countryside walk as being 'the best', when it comes to wellbeing, all sorts of environments, both built and rural, can enhance aspects of our mental health. In fact, regularly walks around local town streets can be nurturing if they are associated with good times.

Walking can also lead to an increase in social capital and social networks, which in turn may have a positive effect on mental well-being. A couple of years ago, I organised a group walk in a local park on Saturday mornings. Each week a few more people came along, to meander through the fairly wild setting and have a cup of tea after the walk. Although this sounds fairly humble, the knock on effects just snowballed. Firstly, people took to cleaning up bits and pieces from the park, and then some of the group decided that they would help in an orchard project that they stumbled upon in the course of the walk and various people became friends and sorted out each others' lives by the looks of things. The really big win though, was talk of a theatrical arts group. All this in a not too affluent area of Birmingham! It all started with walking.

Volunteer-run groups all over the world organise regular walks and even more meditative or solution-focused walks where people are encouraged to use their surroundings as inspiration. Bringing people together in this way is a very strong indicator of the power of walking in terms of strengthening communities and society.

Psychological wellbeing involves the way we feel day to day and being able to deal with periods of mental ill health, including issues like depression and anxiety. Thankfully, we can now speak openly about these common health issues that impact the lives of so many people. Physical activity has long been associated with helping to alleviate the symptoms of depression and anxiety, in fact, for a long time now exercise has been recognised to be as useful as drugs in some cases, leading to the provision of 'exercise on prescription'. People treated with exercise can have lower relapse rates than those treated with medication therapy alone (Phillips et al., 2003).

It seems that regular exercise may make you less likely to become ill in the first place. Numerous studies have shown that people who do a moderate amount of exercise are less likely to suffer depression in the medium term. I feel that this is particularly the case with walking as it may contribute to positive development in terms of both relaxation and resilience, something that more strenuous exercise is less likely to do.

Of course, individual circumstances mean that it is less likely for some groups of people to be exercising regularly than others, this includes people with poor mental health in the first place, or chronic physical health conditions. If you have an illness such as cancer or diabetes you may also be less able to do many types of exercise and this may make your mental health worse. Once again, this is where walking comes into its own: it is a form of exercise that people with pre-existing health conditions (after a professional medical assessment) can, in the main, safely participate in. The accessibility of walking is what makes it such a great asset for psychological health. When you are not feeling great the last thing many people want to do is go to any effort. Most exercise takes preparation time and effort, for example to get kit ready, go to a venue, meet other team members or participants (when you may not want to mix with other people who might seem to have little understanding of the way you are feeling). Not so walking. Walking is an exercise that is as easy as opening your door and taking the first steps outside, with encouragement and support if needed.

Walking, anecdotally, has since the beginning of time been a companion to reflection and letting off steam. In communities across the globe people automatically seem to know that walking will make them feel. People who walk regularly do this not so much because they are thinking about how it is going to improve their blood sugar levels or their blood pressure responses: they do it because they enjoy the feeling of wellbeing that comes with walking.

Becoming and staying a walker helps with depression, anxiety, mood disorders and ADHD, the sort of issues that are sadly increasingly common nowadays as a result of more uncertainty coupled with the negative effects of some elements of normal life such as social media and increasing social tensions. We are not going to change the way the world works around us (at least not overnight) but we can strengthen our ability to deal effectively with life and take some control of our psychological health.

In today's world we are at the mercy of factors that all appear to militate against our mental health and seem to drive anxiety or make us feel depressed. Being uncertain of things naturally makes us anxious and we don't live in a very certain world right now. When we communicate less and less in authentic 'human' ways we may be adding stresses that we are not aware of at a conscious level. The societies we live in are increasingly confusing. There are expectations that we project a particular positive and optimistic image of ourselves that conforms to the narrative that we remain upbeat butthere is plenty of evidence staring us in the face that things are tough and getting tougher for many people, or that the bubble might burst at any time if you are one of the 'winners' in the casino-like world we live in.

In the face of all this, walking can be a powerful treatment for depression and anxiety. The mechanisms for this are not clear because, as we all know, the mind is very complicated and, even now, not that well understood. The mechanisms could involve neural networks firing more effectively and in new patterns, or the reduction of harmful changes in the brain such as inflammation. Positive chemicals like endorphins, and oxytocin (the chemicals that lift our spirits and make us feel good and secure) could also be boosted by walking. Physical activity immediately boosts the brain's dopamine, norepinephrine, and serotonin levels — all of which affect focus and attention. In this way, exercise works in much the same way as ADHD medications such as Ritalin and Adderall. An exercise-induced increase in blood circulation to the brain helps to keep us alert and able to react to situations rationally. Studies show that thirty minutes of exercise of moderate intensity, such as brisk walking for three days a week, is sufficient to reduce anxiety and tension. Moreover, these thirty minutes need not to be continuous; three ten minute walks are believed to be as equally useful as one thirty minute walk.

Walking may also be a tool for people recovering from addictions or trauma. It is only recently that professionals have begun to understand how walking helps people to conquer addictions and walking therapy for addiction has started to be offered in centres around the world. Early research shows that brisk walking, in common with other exercise, alters dopamine signalling in the brain in ways that may make addictive substances and behaviours less appealing or rewarding. Although this is a new area of research, people have instinctively turned to walking as a way to deal with addiction for a very long time. It seems that people intuitively find it helpful to go for regular, often long, walks at a brisk pace. I imagine that a combination of distracting oneself from the addictive substance or behaviour at large, combined with the meditative nature of walking contributes to the therapeutic power of walking. In terms of smoking, a very common but hard to combat addiction, walking has been shown to reduce both cravings and withdrawal symptoms (Taylor & Katomeri, 2007). Walking both provides a healthy alternative to harmful substances or behaviours and may play a part in reconfiguring the signals and brain chemistry involved in addiction. Just as with illnesses such as depression, walking is a safe activity that could be used alongside medical treatments for addiction.

There are other less easy to quantify but equally important factors that may provide an answer as to why walking makes a positive difference to our psychological health. We all know the feeling of being burdened by over-thinking, especially when we can't seem to stop going over and over the same negative interpretation of a part of our lives, or a decision that we came to regret. I know that this is something that I frequently used to do about life decisions: thoughts going round and round my head until I felt worn out by this. Walking, with its ability to help you 'zone-out' of persistent thoughts is a way to distract yourself from negative thinking and focus more on just feeling yourself glide along. You feel that your mind empties itself of rubbish and just drifts. This can be very useful in giving you the rest you need from the thoughts that may be driving depression or anxiety: breaking the cycle, so to speak.

The very act of walking brings a degree of certainty that combats the uncertainty that drives anxiety. Putting one foot in front of the other: we know what that feels like. As we move forward we gather a simple form of confidence and security from this most basic of actions that, unlike everything around us, does not change and is reliable. This has a calming effect on the mind. It also has a positive effect on the body. Quite apart from the improvements to physical health that I outlined in the last chapter, walking seems to alleviate the physical symptoms of stress in real-time: relaxing knotted up muscles and calming down anxiety-induced rapid breathing for example. Just breaking the cycle of these symptoms can have a vastly positive impact on psychological health.

It is the almost meditative nature of walking that may, for many people, be so helpful. This is reflected in outcomes such as feeling the sense of time pressure drop away whilst on a walk. Many of us feel extremely tense about time on a daily basis, commuting, meetings and appointments all contribute to the pressure, so countering this may help to make a real difference to our stress levels. I suggest that you don't keep checking the time when you walk — or even how far you have walked; this might not be easy to start with but the freedom from checking information every few seconds on your phone will be worth it.

Other aspects of psychological health have also been found to measurably increase as a result of regular walking, including hard to define outcomes such as a sense of personal growth (more on this later).

Walking is good for our mental health, but are some walks better than others? Is walking alone best, or with friends? Should you be doing one big walk or spreading your walking throughout the day? Is there a particular secret to the way you walk that might have a bearing on how much of an impact walking will have? Is urban walking just as good for you as walking in the countryside, or in a forest? Let me try and answer some of these questions.

Walking with other people is a way to socialise, as well as to exercise. Furthermore, it is a type of socialising that is becoming increasingly rare: face to face interaction. Make no mistake; we are social animals that need to communicate. When people are deprived of the opportunity to interact, it is devastating for our mental health. It is with good reason that solitary confinement is the ultimate sanction in prisons. Even if we think of ourselves as 'loners' our mental health deteriorates given extended periods without communicating with other people. So, if you spend a lot of time on your own, walking with others provides the balance that we need in terms of companionship. Other people have hectic lives and plenty of company and would possibly welcome a bit of time on their own. The upshot is that there is no definitive answer to the question of whether to walk on your own or with company; it depends on the person and the situation. There are times when it is good to walk alone, when taking a calming walk through a park for example. Meditative walks may be best done alone. Resilience and self-reliance may be encouraged by lone walking. On the other hand, studies have shown that we tend to feel more revitalised by walking when we are in the company of friends. The social context of a walk matters. This is why walking groups are such a good thing and why people are more likely to continue to walk long-tem once they are part of a group (Johansson et al., 2011).

Walking with one other person brings other subtle benefits to communication. During a walk people generally stand side by side. This makes walking and talking a lot less intimidating since it lacks the confrontational positioning that facing head-on would have. Therefore, walking alongside someone is a great way to have a conversation about sensitive issues that you might feel a bit awkward about. Unfortunately, people are also becoming less used to talking 'in real life', which can lead to embarrassment as they struggle to find the words and avoid eye contact in real-world situations rather than online. In my view, this very sad state of affairs can be arrested by using walking as the first step towards reclaiming the ability to talk with people face to face in a fluid way. Walking without directly looking at someone avoids the stress that some people have, for example, when facing a companion at a table or desk.

During a walk people find it easier to drift from one conversation to another. This may be due to a relationship between the cadence of the walk and talk and being in harmony with the surroundings. As the environment around you changes, for example in terms of moving from a track to a road, or a forest to a hill, it somehow becomes easier to change conversation topic without this appearing out of place or rude. Handy obstacles like gates or crossings also give an opportunity to move on from conversation that may be getting stressful, or, indeed, boring.

Periods of silence are another accepted part of walking. Whereas if you were sitting in a room with someone, being quiet may seem rather odd, this is not the case when walking. The concept of 'thinking-time' is at home on a walk, even if you are walking with others. This natural experience of 'breaks' in the flow of a dialogue is a feature of walking and talking that adds value to the activity and is a useful way of learning how to use time to think and reflect or just to take time out of talking to allow your mind to suggest ideas and options to you at either a conscious or subconscious level.

This brings me to the classification of walking in terms of its therapeutic nature as either 'athletic', 'leisure' or 'meditative'. There are crossovers between these types of walk. For example, an athletic walk can also be a leisure walk for many people and a leisure walk can also be meditative. On the whole though, athletic walks are the brisker walks that tend to have the most impact on your physical health and result in physical health outcomes such as improving the ability to control your blood sugar. Leisure walks tend to have the most impact on your happiness derived from being with other people and, indeed, leisure walking can also be very helpful in terms of gaining confidence and resilience and I'll be looking at this later in this book. Leisure walks don't have to be with others though: many people love the opportunity to spend some time walking on their own, getting away from the interference of other people in their lives for a while. The third type of walking, meditative walking, is one that I feel has enormous potential in terms of psychological wellbeing. It is inextricably linked with the concept of mindfulness and also with notions such as 'forest bathing'. In other words, meditative walking is something pictured as being done in a green environment. I agree that the ideal environment to walk in for psychological benefit is a natural one, however I don't feel that you *have* to be in the countryside to benefit, neither do I feel that an athletic type walk cannot be meditative: it just depends on the person.

Walking can be an ideal way to deal with stressful situations before they get out of control. Anecdotally, many of us know the feeling of using a walk to calm down or get our thoughts in order. It seems that this is not just in our imagination as this calming effect has been proved in studies. Young adults who walked for fifty minutes in nature after a stressful situation showed reduced stress and anger and increased positive affect. This relaxing effect, in my view, has a place in terms of anger management and emotional support (Bang et al., 2017, p. 728).

The last element I want to look at in terms of psychological benefits is the additional benefits a walk can bring as a counter to the negative psychological impact of our social-media and digitally obsessed lifestyle. It is a fact of life that we spend much of our time online, either sitting in front of a screen or looking down at one that we are holding. The long-term impact of living in this way is yet to be known but after a relatively small number of years with this being the norm, we can already see many negative outcomes. Physically, a digitally oriented life brings a myriad of problems from poor posture to the cardiovascular and metabolic problems I've already referred to. Of course, sitting for much of the time also makes people more prone to weight-gain and its associated problems too. Looking at screens, especially on mobiles, for a large part of the day can also have an impact on eye strain. Games played online or on a console generally do not have the same positive effect on physical or psychological health as games played in real life and, despite the attempts of major technology companies to marry gaming with exercise, moving in front of a screen is generally no substitute for the range of movement people have access to with traditional sports, or, indeed, walking. In addition, the best environment for any form of exercise in terms of boosting wellbeing is the outdoors and specifically environments that are high on bio-diversity: which most people's living rooms are not!

We are all now dependent on communicating digitally. The always-on, social media led environment which we inhabit brings a stream of negative consequences for our mental health. So, for example, we increasingly view ourselves through the lens of other people's social media responses and become anxious if we don't get the feedback that we expect. Round the clock information leaves us in a state of heightened anticipation and even fear, which social media ruthlessly exploits. We tend to lose our perspective in such an environment and panic or become mildly depressed about situations over which we have little or no control. Being part of an online world brings plenty of benefits in terms of connectivity to other people but it also means that we don't actually communicate face to face much and this has a knock on effect in terms of our confidence with other people. As more and more of our sensory stimuli come from screens we are fooled into believing that we need constant stream of high-octane action to fulfil us. Social media influencers dominate lives and prescribe what to like and what not to like. Many of us self-determine our identity from our online, rather than out real-life presence.

These trends have been heavily reinforced with the onset of Covid-19. Globally, people have had no alternative but to become even more dependent on the online world, in fact working, education and socialising became almost exclusively online. Whilst some people warmed to this, many hated the feeling of entrapment that being under lockdown meant. Through this experience, my understanding of the power of walking increased. Walking gives an opportunity to break free of the 'half-world' that we inhabit when we spend so much of our time on-screen.

Leaving your phone at home (or in your pocket if you are not quite ready to break the chain) means that you instantly become more responsible for living in the real world. Yes, it will feel scary at first but it is worth the initial separation anxiety to feel human again. Walking outdoors enables people to connect with the real world in the most tangible way possible. You are literally grounded in reality. Taking time away from social media means that you begin to realise just how nonsensical it is to depend on this for external validation. Instead you start to gain an appreciation of the importance of your own your own actions and interactions.

The act of walking itself is something that you have to do independently: no one else will do it for you. So you start to gain confidence in your own ability from the start of your walking experience. Walking then becomes an adventure in which you start to intuitively feel connected with your surroundings and more content in yourself. This transition does not depend on being in a green environment but being in nature does provide a sharp contrast to the unreality of the online world and this has a massively positive impact on people. If you walk with other people, walking gives an opportunity to learn (or relearn) the skills that are lost when you don't physically talk to people, especially at a discussion level. People learn the ropes of forming an argument, listening and understanding cues in conversation that are missing in online communication and, as walking provides a low-tension vehicle for talking it is an enjoyable way to find out just how much better life is in the real world.

The move to home working during and post lockdown makes integrating walking into daily routines even more important for both physical and psychological reasons. Transitioning from having an external workplace to home-working has been a rollercoaster experience for many people around the world. To start with, people welcomed the move to home-working as it meant the absence of commuting and the relief of not having people in as close control of one's work. However, without the need to even walk across a car-park or to different parts of an office building, working from home brought a litany of potential health problems for some people. The need to be always available meant that many people felt compelled to be sitting at a desk, whereas they may have been 'around' an office or other workplace. As explained before, constant sitting brings problems for your body: muscles weaken, backs and shoulders hunch and circulation gets worse. Sitting also brings problems for your digestive system, which, for some, was already overloaded by the frequent visits made to the fridge, which became scarily handy for people as they working from home.

Then there is the impact on sleep. Some people found it hard to sleep, whilst others had no problem sleeping but experienced one of the most distressing side effects of the Covid era: vivid dreams, sometimes of a frightening nature. Dreams are full of symbolism and are felt to reflect real the emotions that we feel during our waking hours, so it is hardly surprising that people's dreams included bugs, zombies and all manner of Coronavirus metaphors.

In one sense even bad dreams are a good thing, since dreams allow us to work things out in our subconscious so that we can deal with issues when we are awake, however if nightmares become frequent then we can actually become stressed by the dreams themselves.

So, how can walking help? Firstly, walking has been proven to help us get to sleep and sleep more soundly throughout the night. This may be due to the fact that walking has a positive effect on the regulation of the immune-inflammatory response, core body temperature, autonomic function, and endocrine function, as well as through psychological pathways, such as the improvement of mood. It's been shown that forest walking is helpful for improving sleep and it seems that the afternoon is the best time to take a walk to ensure that you sleep well (Morita et al., 2011). Going for a walk may be an accessible and cost-effective approach for managing sleep problems, whether in lockdown or at any other time. What of the more general psychological impact of working from home: can walking help?

Working from home has meant that many of us now rely increasingly on apps like Zoom and Skype for our work communication, rather than face to face interaction. The repercussions of this are not known, but already many people are feeling the strain of not having access to actual people with whom to communicate. Work is not just 'work', it is also a social experience; the human contact you have with other people 'in the flesh' is valuable in itself. For this reason (and because contact with other people is limited anyway during lockdown), walking may provide a safety net that allows people to generate valuable human interaction under this new way of working.

Since working from home is to set to permanently replace many in-office settings, walking may be critical to maintaining wellbeing. In my view, walking provides a flexible solution to work from home health issues. Walking on your own mitigates the physical health issues and, perhaps surprisingly, even provides a degree of social contact that is extremely important in a work from home scenario. A regular walk around a park, for example, means that you may see more or less the same people every time you go and this familiarity may result in at least an innate acknowledgement, if not a small exchange of glances saying 'hello fellow walker' ,or over time, a friendly hello and a chat. The human contact brought about by this simple act of sharing a common interest with people who become familiar might, in the future make home working more tolerable and interesting.

In my view, 'away from desk' experiences need to be built into the work from home day. Walking in a group (even if socially distanced during the Covid-19 period) may bring different benefits of reinforcing communication skills and a feeling of being part of a team (even if not your own work team but another self-selected group with common interest). The move to working from home has changed from being a temporary way to cope with a crisis, to becoming a permanent feature of business and work, with companies such as Fujitsu and Facebook announcing that some of their teams will be permanently working from home. I do feel that companies have underestimated the human need for companionship beyond seeing a figure on a screen: walking programmes provide a way for people to maintain their physical and psychological health in the work from home era.

To summarise some main points relating to walking and psychological wellbeing:

- Psychological health problems have become more prevalent in recent years due to increasing uncertainty, increasing inequality and rapid change. Walking is an accessible form of exercise that has been shown to reduce anxiety and depression, in some cases as effectively as medication.

- People have instinctively walked as a way to deal with stress for millennia. Walking has also traditionally been used as a way to unwind and recharge.

- Walking is an effective way to distract oneself from negative thoughts and improve attention. This may make it a valuable tool in terms of dealing with issues like ADHD and anger management. Walking enables you to enter into a calmer semi-meditative state that gives your mind a break from over-thinking.

- Mindful walking and meditative walking are effective ways to reduce stress, particularly in green spaces. This entails letting go of negative thoughts and taking in one's surroundings and having a quiet awareness of oneself. The most therapeutic environments for walking are forests and near natural water.

- Poor sleep leads to a multitude of health problems. Walking can help people sleep better.

- Smoking and other addictions may be controlled by walking, which could both reduce cravings and help with withdrawal symptoms

- As people spend more time online, walking is a valuable way to connect with the real world in a tangible way. This has numerous benefits including enabling people to assess issues more effectively and connect with people in real life.

- Walking is a low-stress way to communicate with other people, which improves social wellbeing and reduces loneliness. Working from home can leave people feeling isolated and shut in. Walking is a way to mitigate this.

There is plenty to recommend walking as a strong tool to help with mental health issues and general psychological wellbeing. Walking around your neighbourhood will bring these benefits for most people. What if you could boost the positive benefits even more? There is one proven way to make your walks even better for you — walking in green and natural surroundings.

At Walking Pace

Green Walking

Before I think about the benefits of green walking I want to
turn to mindfulness and its use as part of the walking
experience. Mindfulness is a fairly new concept that many
walkers have traditionally incorporated into their walking
without labelling it as such. I am pretty sure that, when
walking was a bigger part of people lives in the historical or
pre-historical past, people practiced mindfulness when they
walked; they just didn't give it a label. Mindfulness relates to
being 'mindful' of the entire experience you are in, at the
moment you are experiencing it. This incorporates your
thoughts and feelings as well as your surroundings. So, this
includes being aware of your own breathing say, or the way
that the ground feels under your feet, or the movement of the
air around you. As you fill your consciousness with the
movement of your body, your breathing and the world
directly around you, you can let go of worries running
through your head and even, over time, lose the harmful
feelings associated with trauma or issues like obsessive
compulsive disorder. This awareness is felt to ground people
in reality, rather than leave them in their previous state of
being fixated on persistent negative thinking about the past

or future (in this respect it is similar to cognitive behavioural therapy) and it is felt to have a calming effect psychologically. Mindfulness is therefore a pragmatic way to focus on appreciating the here and now and to be proactive about life, since these are traits that I value highly I certainly feel that mindfulness can be a very helpful element of walking and vice versa.

Mindful walks tend to be slow and deliberate, allowing the walker to take in the surroundings properly but there is no reason, in my view, why mindfulness should not extend to a brisker walk. Brisk walking has a different and complementary function when it comes to psychological health. As the walking tempo increases blood flow it also creates a feeling of alertness that is known scientifically as 'activation'. Activation may be enhanced by being mindful and, coupled with the improved physical outcomes of brisk walking, leads to a feeling of wellbeing.

I want now to turn to something that has gained a lot of interest in recent years and has been the subject of many research studies, the vast majority of which point to the same outcome: walking in green space is good for your psychological wellbeing.

Just being in nature is good for you: it doesn't matter what you are doing in them — natural environments enhance wellbeing. Even having access to a view of countryside out of a window, without actually going outside, helps people feel better and has a real effect positive effect on your blood pressure. It is thought that we soak up positive stimuli from being in green and peaceful surroundings, which cause us to redirect our attention away for negative thoughts.

As opposed to the urban environment, we almost universally think of the countryside as being 'restorative' and this has been the case since we started living in cities: just consider all those Victorians who used to take the air in spa towns or on the coast. Long before mindfulness was a thing, being in a green place was felt to improve wellbeing by being away from energy sapping activities and replacing these with the involuntary attention we can't help but give to the little things happening around us in the countryside: the flow of a stream or the movement of the trees for example. Of course the restorative value will depend on a few other variables such as whether we feel that we have the time to spend in our green environment (if we can't stop thinking that we should be somewhere else then the benefits will be more limited). All things being equal however, it seems that attention does improve significantly when you head outside and walk, leading to a case to be made to reduce the pills and increase the outdoor adventure. In the attention-compromised world around us, we should be looking to latch onto activities and environments that help us to concentrate and focus. The combination of walking and a green environment does exactly that.

The Covid-19 crisis made us all aware of the downside of living in densely populated areas, and the relative freedom of being in the countryside. Away from the city one could go about without having to dodge other people in order to socially distance. This, when combined with the instinctive sense of wellbeing derived from being in green spaces and an increase in working from home has led to a drift from city to countryside living.

Of course, 'country walking' can mean very different things to different people. In one case, walking could be interpreted as a long-hill hike and in another case a stroll through a meadow. It doesn't matter: being outside and walking is good for you regardless. Let's take an example that is pretty much middle of the road: a walk with a few people in a relatively unknown location with a bit of adventure thrown in by way of finding different places. This sort of walking experience brings psychological benefits by way of, firstly, gaining a sense of freedom and escape. This is an intangible but real attribute of walking: you can walk pretty much where your legs can carry you. For people tied to an office desk just the pure feeling of being able to 'breathe' is an important factor in green walking. This is allied to another benefit: being in tune with nature and gaining sensitivity to your environment. This creates a sense of shared ownership and responsibility for our surroundings that enhances our enjoyment. By walking in green spaces, which are much bigger in scale than the rooms and streets we spend much of our time in we can physically gain a sense of perspective. Look up through the treetops at the sky when walking through a forest and you immediately feel a sense of being part of a bigger picture and this helps you to see any issues in a different way.

So, what of actual, researched comparisons between walks in urban areas and walks in green or blue (next to water) areas? Many studies have shown that walking in areas such as forests have more positive effects on physical and psychological health than walking in the city. This has led to the coining of phrases such as 'forest therapy', credited with beneficial effects such as lowering blood pressure and improving the body's response to infection. Forest walking has also been shown to significantly increase people's positive emotions and decrease their negative emotions compared with activities in urban areas (Song et al., 2018)

The benefits of green walking have been popularised with a trend towards forest bathing or shinrin-yoku, a phenomenon that originated in Japan in the 1980s as an antidote to the oppressive urban living conditions of Japanese city dwellers. As more research highlighted the benefits of shinrin-yoku, the Japanese government incorporated it into the country's health programme. The practice, which combines being in a calm forest environment combined with a quiet awareness of oneself and the surroundings has been shown to reduce blood pressure, lower cortisol levels and improve concentration and memory. A chemical released by trees and plants, called phytoncides, has been shown to boost the immune system, which could partially explain why walking though forest environments is good for us, coupled with the calming effect of a peaceful environment. Studies have found that forest environments help people experiencing chronic stress. So, forest-bathing may be suitable as a stress reduction tool, and forests can be viewed as therapeutic landscapes (Morita et al., 2007).

Let's look at some fairly commonsense observations. Walking on your own in a natural environment generally makes you feel better than walking indoors or in an urban environment. On top of this, walking in a maintained forest has a more beneficial effect than walking in a wild unmaintained forest. If you, like me, have threaded your way through brambles and over fallen logs you will understand why, for most people, a secure forest path is a preferable walking area (although I like the challenge of a mini-adventure through the wilderness it must be said). Walking on your own in green spaces is more likely to reduce negative emotions and stress when compared to walking alone in urban environments.

Group walks, however, bring other benefits in terms of social health and wellbeing (for example in terms of self-esteem) and group walks in natural environments can have an effect on well-being greater than either just the act of walking or just the social environment. Previous research suggests that feelings of restoration from natural environments may be diminished when walking with others. For example, the effects of psychological restoration from walking in a nature setting are greater when alone than with others — but only if you feel safe. Conversely, feelings of revitalization are greater when walking in an urban environment with a friend compared to walking alone in an urban environment (Johansson et al., 2011). Of course, the benefits of walking on your own, or with other people will depend on the type of person that you are and what specific outcome you would like to gain from the walking experience at any one time.

Studies show that there is a hierarchy of natural environments. Even though being in nature is better on the whole than being in the city, it seems that some environments are better for your psychological health than others. It figures that walking in these higher ranking environments is going to be better for your wellbeing. Farmland, woodland and grassland are all good to walk in but for an even greater lift in psychological wellbeing, forests and aquatic areas are in top place. Indeed, a "blue" gradient in health and mental health has been found, in which self-reported physical and mental health improves the closer an individual lives to the sea, over and above the effects of green environments. Walking near water leads to even greater improvements in self-esteem and mood compared to exercising in urban green space, farmland and woodland environments (Pasanen TP et al., 2019).

So, what about walking in the city, but in a park or garden? It seems that in a city the more 'natural' the area we walk in, the greater the benefit to mental health and wellbeing. This might be because of the amount of biodiversity, such as number of plant species and habitat types. But just being in any green corridor, be this garden, park or country-park may be a protective factor against the negative effects of the stresses of today (Duvivier, 2020). Indeed, given that walking per se has a positive effect on psychological wellbeing, no matter where you do it, it follows that walking, combined with the added psychological benefits of being in nature, will be even more beneficial to one's psychological health. So, if you live in a city and don't have great access to the countryside you can still gain the benefits of 'green-walking' by striding out in a local park or green corridor. If you have a canal or a river running through your town then walking alongside this will lift your spirits and wellbeing.

Walking has re-emerged as a natural tonic for the mind. Techniques such as mindfulness and forest bathing are a nod to the spiritual knowledge of ancient people who recognised the power of walking for psychological wellbeing. This aspect of walking further elevates the role of walking in terms of improving general health. This begs the question: could walking actually keep you young? In the next chapter I look at the role of walking as an antidote to a couple of the health issues we meet in later life.

At Walking Pace

Can Walking Keep You Young?

As the human lifespan becomes longer, sadly it don't necessarily become healthier. More years yes, but sometimes more years to fear losing our independence, social lives and our health. Amongst the biggest of our fears is the possibility that we might develop dementia: a progressive condition that has symptoms that includes memory loss and difficulties with thinking, problem-solving or language. The most common form of dementia is Alzheimer's disease, which we associate with confusion and profound memory loss.

Retiring from work can sometimes mean that we feel lonelier and bored because we lose a sense of purpose and the companionship and routine of the workplace; this can lead to mental ill health such as depression. The feeling of being superfluous to requirements can be made worse by the realisation that society tends to value young people more than those who are getting on a bit and sometimes dehumanises older people and makes them 'invisible'.

Major physical health problems in middle-age are exacerbated by the weight gain that many people experience at this time. Joint problems such as arthritis, cardio-vascular problems and respiratory illness are just some of the health issues that are much more common in the second half of our lives. I will focus on just a couple of these health issues in this chapter and explain how becoming fitter helps us all to age in a healthier, happier way. The changes that occur with ageing are complex and, of course there is no holy grail of eternal youth, however, there is a growing body of evidence that suggests that walking could be a useful weapon against some of the effects of aging — in middle-age and beyond.

The physical health benefits of walking, such as maintaining a healthy weight are undoubtedly a way to stay fitter as we grow older. Mid-life is when most people are at their heaviest, in fact approaching 50 percent of middle-aged adults aged 40 to 59 years are classed as obese in the US (*CDC*, 2020). Although usually gaining less media attention than weight gain earlier in life, a very significant proportion of people over the age of 60 are overweight in developed countries (approximately 70 percent in the US) This makes people more prone to diseases such as diabetes, cardio-vascular disease, cancer and bone joint problems such as osteoporosis. Obesity also raises the risk of severe problems when associated with other illnesses (such as with Covid-19). Being significantly overweight makes the risk of dying from weight-related disease greater for older people. The lungs of obese patients decrease in size, making it easier to develop respiratory problems such as pneumonia, which are more common in later life anyway because immunity decreases with age.

The reasons that older people seem to gain weight more easily are multi-faceted and include physiological, hormonal and environmental changes. As we grow older muscle mass decreases and fat mass increases; lower muscle mass makes it more difficult to walk with the ease we used to when we were young. This leads to less physical movement and, when accompanied by not cutting back on food, a net calorie excess, which, of course, means getting fatter. Hormonal and metabolic changes also make us more prone to being overweight. For example we develop a resistance to leptin, a protein hormone that regulates energy intake and expenditure. It's also believed that aging plays a role in reduced responsiveness to thyroid hormone and, as we age, our digestive systems work less efficiently, which means less energy from food is burned off as calories while more is stored as fat; as a result we gain weight more quickly and lose weight more slowly.

So, maintaining a healthy weight is extremely important later in life and exercise is a key component in this. Yet the types of exercise people used to do when younger may not travel very well into later years. The reality is that mountain biking, running and other high impact sports are going to be ruled out for most people as our bodies lose power when we grow older and our increased susceptibility to injury makes it less enjoyable and more risky to participate in these activities. Older people may also feel uncomfortable in gyms or sporting venues which are marketed heavily towards younger customers.

Fortunately, weight gain into older years is not inevitable and walking can play a big part in weight maintenance for all of us through the years — a part that extends way beyond just calories burnt. As described earlier, regular walkers put on less weight over time, so starting walking and keeping walking will make it less likely that you will have a weight problem when older. However, it is never too late to start walking to improve your overall health.

Walking is a flexible activity. Even if you are completely unused to exercise per se most of us walk to some degree, even if this is just pottering around the house. For someone nervous about exercising, the fact that walking can be done in the home is a secure way of starting to improve physical health. Further walking can be slowly built up over time: remember that three ten minute walks are as beneficial to health as one thirty minute walk. Walking is a great way to preserve muscle and bone mass, leading to more confidence with balance and the potential to walk for longer periods of time.

Going for a walk with other people provides the perfect antidote to the isolation that can cause so much harm to mental health in later life. Walking and talking in fact kills two birds with one stone as people gain the companionship and mental stimulation that helps to maintain a positive outlook and sharpen communication skills, whilst also developing community support with others committed to maintaining a healthy lifestyle.

There are therefore real physical health benefits to walking as we grow older. However, the real magic bullet of walking may be in predicting or even slowing the onset of Alzheimer's disease and other forms of dementia. The reasons why people develop cognitive disorders such as dementia are complex and uncertain but it seems that a reduction in blood flow to the brain may be one factor. As already discussed, replacing sitting with walking helps to speed up blood flow in people of all ages.

Dementia is a major reason for disability and shortening of life for older people. It has a devastating impact on quality of life therefore identifying ways to detect or slow down dementia is very important in order to preserve the quality of life of people as they age. Dementia develops slowly for many people and any clues to its progression that can be measured could be very useful in starting early treatment. For some time now, there has been a link made between walking and dementia in that people with a faster walking speed have been shown to be statistically less likely to develop dementia (Hackett et al., 2018).

A slowing in walking speed has also been shown to increase the risk of dementia. People aged over sixty whose walking speed fell most over as short a period as a couple of years are more likely to develop dementia according to the English Longitudinal Study of Ageing. This relationship was found regardless of the original walking speed. So, someone whose walking speed slows down rapidly could be at greater risk of developing dementia. Of course this is not to say that a slower walking speed causes dementia but the link between walking and the cognitive decline associated with dementia is real and interesting.

It may be that walking speed and dementia are linked because walking and cognition both rely on similar brain regions in the prefrontal cortex of the brain and as changes in these parts of the brain happen they affect both walking speed and also cognition. Inflammation of the brain can also affect the 'neuro-plasticity' of the brain and also muscle strength — another possible connection between walking speed and cognition. Finally, issues that affect blood flow (vascular) health of the brain such as stroke and general cardiovascular health may also provide the link between walking and dementia risk. Unfortunately, slow walking is not just associated with dementia; it is also associated with many other health problems that limit our lifespan and quality of life including heart problems and slow recovery from diseases in general. Neither is the link just confined to old age; it has recently been discovered that 'gait speed' is an indicator of health problems even in middle-age and probably even earlier in life (Rasmussen et al., 2019). It seems that walking speed really matters.

So, if slow walking can predict an increased likelihood to develop dementia, could it be that speeding up your walking, through increased and regular walking activity can reduce your likelihood of developing dementia? There is not enough evidence out there at present to definitively say this yet but walking does have a positive impact on the issues that I've outlined as being relevant to brain health including blood flow and inflammation. Evidence that walking exercises do have a positive effect on cognitive function for people with dementia is also starting to emerge. Research has shown that exercise in general has a beneficial effect on cognition. Researchers from the University of California found that people actively suffering from Alzheimer's disease who did more than two hours of walking a week had a significant improvement in both their cognition and mood. The researchers showed that walking regularly every week could actually stabilise Alzheimer's disease over the course of a year (Winchester et al., 2013).

Yet another study found that fifteen weeks of physical activity comprised of three one hour sessions of walking per week improved cognitive functions for people with dementia, compared to people who did not walk (whose pace and stride length actually decreased). This study showed that a physical activity programme can slow cognitive decline and improve quality of walking in elderly people suffering from dementia (Kemoun et al., 2010). Furthermore, walking seems to have a positive impact on the level of depression people with dementia suffer (C. L. Williams & Tappen, 2008).

Since improved memory performance has been found to be linked to walking as well (Cavalcante et al., 2018), it seems that walking is a suitable way for older people to exercise in order to maintain the best natural defence against dementia. Walking also brings the additional benefits of enhancing overall health and, in particular, is a safe and accessible way to maintain a healthy weight in older age. Walking in a group enhances social links and walking conversations do a lot to keep the mind active. You won't be surprised to learn that I am a big advocate of walking for older people.

I have outlined the place of walking in mitigating two significant health risks we face as we grow older: obesity and dementia. There are many other ways that walking keeps us young, including making us feel positive about life and the changes it brings over time.

Having seen how walking can bring big gains in terms of physical and mental health and how it can potentially extend and improve our later years, I want to turn to how walking can influence wellbeing in terms of how we think creatively and the subsequent impact it has had because of this. In the next short section, I'll look at how walking has played a role in creativity and culture for hundreds of years and how it is has a great many artistic fans. Ideas need creativity and work needs ideas, so a natural progression of the value of walking is its potential to contribute to innovation at work.

At Walking Pace

Art and Walking

There is no universal definition of creativity, but a common definition outlines a creative idea as being novel or original as well as useful, adaptive, or functional. It is the first criteria that applies to the 'arts' and the second criteria that applies more to problem-solving and work (more of which later). Taken together, the two dimensions of creativity play an enormous part in shaping personal and societal development.

Earlier in this book I described how writers and philosophers though the ages have used walking to generate their ideas. For example, Aristotle, used to give lectures while walking around his school in Athens, followed by his pupils who became known as 'peripatetics' (meaning moving around). Charles Dickens was an avid daily walker who regularly walked twenty to thirty miles a day! Other groups of creatives, including musicians and visual artists have turned to walking to inspire them. Beethoven, for example, relied on daily walking forays for inspiration; during his walks he would continue to write music, scribbled on sheets of music paper that he carried with him.

Visual artists have long been inspired by the landscapes they walked within. Think of any painting by a landscape artist such as Turner and you will instantly feel aware of the walk that they took, ending up at the point that they decided to capture for us. Not only have artists used walking as a way of replenishing their energy and wellbeing, they have actively incorporated the walk as a way to record the world around them, stamping the identity of other walkers within their work. This, to me, is homage to walking itself.

Walking as an integral element of art has a long history. As walkers, artists gain the experience of more fully immersing themselves in their subject matter, or of considering elements such as the political, social or environmental relevance of their work. Walking is now present in art in many different ways: from collective art groups who go on walks, to the long history of political or protest walks that incorporate art forms such as music and banners. Walking and art are intertwined. Indeed walking is a legitimate form of expression in itself. Walking is an 'attitude'.

Members of the Dada art movement in 1920s Paris organised a series of excursions to 'places that have no reason to exist.' Although only one of their nihilistic walks eventually took place, it sounds quite an event: the walk was accompanied by poetry recitals and was performed as a parody of a tour guide, making the walk a piece of performance art itself. A few decades later, artist and philosopher Guy Debord created walking maps highlighting 'psychogeographic contours' through the city, drawing attention to the 'ambience' elicited by different surroundings. His notion of 'derive' saw the city as a living organism, where a walk became a creative experience that generated feelings that could be put to use in any number of ways: from the political to the artistic (Hermon Bashiron Mendolicchio 2020). Thus, walking has long been part of a daringly avant-garde and counter-culture scene.

Some contemporary artists centre their work on walking. They make art where walking is the subject matter: Richard Long's 'A Line made by Walking' photograph, showing a straight line of trampled grass receding towards tall bushes or trees at the far side of what appears to be a field, is a good example. Another is 'walking artist" Hamish Fulton. Since 1973 Fulton has only made works based on the practice of walking, dispensing with what he feels are the materialistic shackles we live with and concentrating on the freedom that walking gives us to think and create. The walk as a symbol of simplicity and an escape from conformity is a well used artistic trope.

Another popular example of 'walking as art' is 'The Lovers', Artists' Marina Abramović and Ulay's 1988 performance, in which they stood 5,995 kilometres apart on the ruins of the Great Wall of China and began walking towards each other. They started from opposite ends: Abramović began from the mountainous provinces of The Yellow Sea while Ulay walked from the Gobi desert. The walk was intended as a metaphor for their love and longing, however it turned into something very different (especially since Ulay had an affair with his translator during the journey) but it was nevertheless interesting, dramatic and thought-provoking.

This association of walking and journeys with discovery and drama is very well exemplified in books and films, indeed there are too many to mention but I'll pick out a couple. The classic 'Wizard of Oz' tells the allegorical story of Dorothy going through Oz 'following the yellow brick road' on a walk with her companions, whilst Cormack McCarthy's 'The Road' offers a disturbing tale of a walk by a father and son though a dystopian post-nuclear destruction America. These two very different stories tap into our deep-seated identification with journeying on foot. The idea of a walk as a means of discovery is deeply embedded within written and visual culture.

Walking then is not a stranger to creative people. Historically, it has been appreciated as a thought and idea-provoking mechanism; walking therefore seems inextricably linked with the creative process. Does research reveal any rationale for walking promoting ideas creation? If indeed walking is a creative force then this opens the door for walking to become a tool, not just for artists but for work that needs people to think of ideas. So, does walking really have a positive effect on creative thinking and, if it does, what could be its greater impact at work?

In the next section, I'll look at the place of walking within the work context, from walking as a means of transport to and from work, to its potential in terms of problem-solving. As work changes dramatically as a result of global events, perhaps now is the time to make walking an accepted part of it?

At Walking Pace

Working and Walking

Work often dominates our lives, so the way that we feel and behave in connection with work is important. Most of us spend a lot of time at work. We can be working in a role where we need to problem-solve intellectually, deal with people, do technical tasks or creative tasks; for many occupations work is a combination of all of these elements. For many of us, work carries with it both rewards and frustrations around getting our jobs done well and with the least amount of stress. We can sometimes struggle with work problems, or feel the heat with workload. Relationships with colleagues can feel strained. The pace of change at work can leave us struggling to understand new ways of doing things, whilst trying to remember how to everything fits together. The shift to working in new ways (such as from home) brings its own challenges.

Work is a major reason why people are sedentary (most people sit down for the majority of their working day) and this creates the risk factors associated with sitting that I've outlined earlier. On a positive note, work can be the ideal arena for positively changing our behaviour.

Organisational strategists spend an awful lot of time (and get paid an awful lot of money) to find better ways to work and to deliver bottom-line results for companies, but could the humble walk play a part in improving work performance and profitability? Over and above the potential to improve physical health, I feel that walking can actually improve our work itself. With this in mind I'll look at the potential for walking to make us sharper, more creative and productive workers.

There are a number of measures that walking may score on that are relevant to work. Walking could be effective in terms of enhancing problem-solving at work, creativity and ideas generation, or just in terms of helping people to feel more relaxed and well. Walking may also have a function in enabling and sustaining healthy communication amongst team members across an organisation. For the increasing number of us working in an isolated way (working from home for an organisation or as a self-employed freelance worker) walking can be a way to engage with other people to fulfil the strong need we have to engage and socialise with others.

Let me start by thinking about an area that is important for most jobs, even if this is not immediately obvious: creativity. Creativity is not just about producing something artistic. It is the act of turning new and imaginative ideas into reality. It is about seeing the world in new imaginative ways, finding hidden patterns and connections between elements that appear unrelated (lateral thinking) and using this insight to generate solutions.

It has been demonstrated that there is a close relationship between creativity and occupational self-efficiency (belief that you can get the job done), as well as healthier psychological functioning, wellbeing, successful adaption to daily changes at work, and better interpersonal relations (Zhou & Hoever, 2014). So, nourishing creativity at work may end up benefitting more than just entrepreneurship or innovation. Work is made up of situations where many of us have to process information, generate ideas and execute actions. As creativity is an indicator of many different work-related skills, enhancing creativity may boost work performance in general.

Walking is felt to have a particular place in encouraging creativity, especially because it encourages divergent thinking: thinking that draws upon ideas from all directions. Divergent thinking, a core process of creativity, leads you to look for options that aren't necessarily apparent at first. Once a problem is defined, divergent thinking is critical for generating innovative, novel, and useful ideas. Given its importance, numerous methods have been developed to enhance divergent thinking such as brainstorming, structured lectures and exercises, social modelling and individualized coaching. Could walking be a novel activity to be added to this list?

Since walking encourages divergent thinking, it is indeed starting to be recognised as an activity feature that could be introduced to the work arena as a catalyst for creativity. The mechanisms for this enhanced creative thinking are not clearly known but one theory is that walking encourages better connections between neural networks, enhancing the brains ability to adapt to different stimuli. Another theory is that walking spreads the activation of neighbouring neural networks, which in turn, may help to facilitate solving a creative solution (Patterson et al., 2018).

Divergent thinking is not just improved during a walk but also afterwards (for example when people get back to the office). Therefore, an after-walk work brainstorming session might be a good ideas generator. Taking different walking routes might make work walks more stimulating and generate different solutions. Walking around local areas of interest and green spaces is a great way to enable divergent, creative ideas but it is walking itself, and not the environment that appears to be the main factor in boosting creative thinking—even walking on a treadmill boosts creativity. Compared to sitting, in fact, creativity can be boosted up to sixty percent when you walk (Oppezzo & Schwartz, 2014). However, it is from a seated position that we are usually tasked with thinking, coming up with ideas and problem-solving. Obviously, it is not practical to be walking about for large parts of the day but some combination of sitting and walking could prove to be a good way to enhance creative problem-solving at work. Work areas that involve discovering new perspectives and ways of doing things such as operations, marketing or communications could benefit from incorporating walking sessions, as could strategic level work where novel solutions to high-level problems are needed.

Divergent thinking, however, is not the only attribute we need at work. We need to think not just divergently but in a focused way, for example to work out calculations or generate a specific answer rather than different options. The benefits of walking to focus are not so clear-cut. Trying to work out the answer to technical problems whilst you are walking might not be that effective. In large scale studies where focused problem solving has been measured at the same time or directly following walking, no advantage has generally been found. This may be because walking actually demands the use of brain power that is also needed for focused thinking; this is not an issue when you are using your mind for divergent thinking but it is an issue when you are trying to actively work on a particular problem. In this scenario, the concentration you devote to solving a mental problem and walking 'interfere' with each other. So, for tasks like creative brainstorming walking is definitely useful, whereas not so much for working out the answer to technical problems needing a specific correct answer. (Al-Yahya et al., 2011).

There is however some evidence that, for people who do want to apply more focus to their walks, there is a particular style of walking that may provide a structured way to bring a walking dividend to concentration and focused problem solving (where there is a crossover of focused and divergent thinking). In a study conducted on academics (in other words people who thought for a living) researchers identified 'walking for thinking' where participants felt that they were able to access their memory and control their cognitive focus as well as generate divergent creative ideas. This required walking with a specific set of characteristics.

The participants all felt that walking for thinking needed a walk with a steady rhythm and a specific individual speed. They felt that walking was a form of 'moving gestalt' with interplay between the person, environment and thinking and the rhythms of the body correlating with the rhythm of walking. Walking, for them, increased their thinking and their awareness. Although this was a limited study it brings insight into the type of walking that could be useful for both walking for creativity and walking for thinking (Keinänen, 2015).

The optimal speed for this type of walking appears to be just less than three miles an hour. Curiously this is the speed at which there is minimal metabolic energy expenditure (when the pelvis, joints and legs are optimally aligned). If you are using your body optimally it makes sense that the mind will benefit by having access to energy, whilst the rest of your body won't be taxed metabolically. Repetitive movement or chanting (as noticed by a host of meditative disciplines) helps focus.

Contrary to the experience of people who seek to soak in their environment or chat to others as they walk, walking for thinking seems most effective when walkers get into the rhythm of walking and don't look to actively process things around them. The tangential intrusion of the surroundings gives just the right amount of stimulation to enhance thinking, without taking over. In this way people avoid 'multi-tasking'. Multi-tasking always reduces thinking capacity, apart from when the other task (alongside thinking) is a simple movement like doodling or walking. Indeed, simple repetitive movement may help in focusing attention rather than distracting it. The world we live in is now full of multi-tasking, especially in terms of using media whist doing other things; having an opportunity to break away from this can encourage effective, focused thinking.

Other research has found that walking appears to have a positive impact on 'cognitive control' (attention) not during walking but afterwards. In fact it was found that a brisk twenty minute walk was an effective way to increase concentration afterwards for young people (Hillman et al., 2009). This could be useful for people with ADHD, or indeed when extra concentration is needed – for example when studying for exams. At work, the idea of taking a walking break and then returning to concentrated work is one that could yield benefits.

Although walking at the optimal speed is not metabolically challenging, it is still fairly aerobic. Aerobic exercise increases blood flow to the brain and reduces stress hormones, this many play a part in stimulating thought processes.

Another brain skill that is essential to work is memory. There is an interesting connection between space, memory and walking. Walking around can help your the mind to remember things more easily. It could be that your subconscious associates where you are with facts and discoveries in an example of interplay between the person, environment and thinking. A well-known memorization technique, the 'method of loci', utilizes this kind of approach through imagery. It relies on imagined spatial relationships to establish order and recollect memories. Using this method you think of a place or route you know well and visualize a series of locations in the place in logical order, you then visualise each item that you want to remember at one of the locations. To remember the items you visualise the route and recall the items as you move along it in your mind. The ability to bring information to the front of your mind when you need it is a key attribute to jobs ranging from carer to scientist. Therefore, increasing walking at work could bring performance dividends in terms of better information recall.

Since integrating walking into one's lifestyle boosts psychological wellbeing in general, the other big work-related issue that walking could help with is wellbeing and psychological welfare at work. This is important as work is potentially where we can feel most stressed. Work often involves time pressures and other stresses related to personal dynamics between colleagues or the frustration of dealing with technology not working effectively. In addition, the inevitable strains of outside work issues spill over into the work domain.

It has been shown that unwinding from job demands (recovery time) is important for reducing the negative effects of work stress. Recovery is different to sleeping: it means returning your body and mind to the state it was in before it became stressed and replenishing depleted energy. In fact, in modern society, which is characterized by a hectic pace of life and unremitting need to be on the go, it is likely that lack of recovery is a very significant health problem. The combination of walking, being away from the work environment and having access to nature can be a big help in recovering from the stresses of work. This recovery may act as a protective mechanism that acts as a buffer at work at times of high pressure and also enables people to be more resilient to work stress in general (de Bloom et al., 2014).

The practice of forest bathing helps with chronic stress, so a mini-version may help with work-related stress issues Walking in a forest may not be the most accessible of pastimes for most of us at work (although if you work near a forest I'm very envious) but a regular walk from a place of work through green space such as a park could give people similar wellbeing benefits. The stress-busting power of green-walking may yet be one of the best defences against work-related stress in these challenging times.

Many of us also associate work with causing us to be in a 'bad-mood' from time to time and work can indeed leave us grumpy and out of sorts. Daily walking has been shown to improve people's mood when compared with not walking. This mood enhancement seems to happen at a deep level and involves mechanisms in our brains triggering a more parasympathetic nervous system response. This is the part of our autonomic nervous system that stops the body from overworking and restores us to a calm and composed state, lowering the heart rate and blood pressure, for example. Although 'mood' is a subjective feeling (what we feel is different for each of us), it seems that walking can lift our spirits and potentially lead to a better experience at work (Sakuragi & Sugiyama, 2006).

A number of companies have started to realise that supporting staff wellbeing is a winner in terms of productivity, reduction in sickness and employee retention. For most of these companies at present, this means improving access to gyms, telehealth (the use of digital information and communication technologies, such as computers and mobile devices, to access health care services remotely and manage health care) and providing courses in activities like yoga. These are all good interventions but corporate wellbeing services could be ignoring offering and promoting the one activity that is accessible, value for money and simple: walking. I am slightly stumped as to why this is but it could be that there are not a great many walk practitioners at present when compared with say yoga or meditation.

Walking could be seen as less 'sexy' than other forms of workplace wellbeing like providing pool tables or relaxation pods. It may also be disadvantaged by being less commercially-oriented: whereas partnerships can be set up between corporates and gym groups for example, such partnerships are less in evidence with walking providers. The weather in some countries (including the UK) may make some people believe that walking is not an activity that can be incorporated into the working day all year round. Of course, walking in the rain might be out for most people but certainly walking in cold but dry weather is an exhilarating experience that brings wellbeing benefits that human-resources departments may not have realised.

Some companies and organisations are genuinely switched on to the issue to being partners in improving the health of employees and to the general consensus that wellbeing needs to be improved in society. As awareness of the dangers of sitting has increased, so more companies have started investigating the potential of standing desks, or even getting small pedal cycles for staff to operate under their desks. Walking or cycling computer work stations are also available. Their investment reflects the fact that some organisations want to play a part in reducing the sitting time of the 70 to 75% of people (in the UK) who extensively use computers in their jobs and therefore spend long periods of time sitting and have low levels of energy expenditure.

To break away from sitting, people need to get up and move around. This is possible if there are other tasks for someone to do that involve leaving the work station, or companies can try and create this 'productive variation' by positioning things people need to do on different floors and encouraging people to walk between these tasks, for example. This, however, is not possible within a lot of workplaces as all work needs to be done statically at a computer. The short breaks of five to ten minutes an hour which are recommended for people who work at a VDU (HSE, 2020) are not actioned or encouraged by organisations in most cases. This is probably because ten minutes per hour in a good chunk out of the entire day and many employers would instinctively see this as losing productive time. In an attempt to find an outwardly less costly solution, the standing desk has become a beneficiary.

Standing desks are all the rage. In fact sales of standing desks in some areas have overtaken those of conventional 'sitting' desks. This has all been prompted by the very real evidence that sitting is bad for our health in terms of obesity, diabetes, cardio-vascular disease and cancer. I am sure that people buying and using standing desks are doing so feeling that they can greatly mitigate their health risks by standing up at work. However not all 'non-sitting' activities are equal. Standing instead of sitting only burns a few more calories an hour, so it has virtually no impact on weight (if you 'reward' yourself for using a standing desk by eating more you could actually put on weight); standing is not an aerobic activity and does not help your cardio-vascular system. Standing without moving much for hours on end can bring additional health problems like developing back, leg, or foot pain or even circulatory problems. Standing for a long time can be uncomfortable for some people and this can reduce concentration, reaction time and even mood...so a standing desk might not be as good for you or your work as manufacturers of standing desks might like to make out.

One step up from standing in the office is the interest in walking and cycling computer workstations. These are treadmills or cycles with spaces for laptops built in and yes, they do burn more calories than just sitting at a desk. The problem with using exercise work stations is that people tend to overestimate just how energetic they are on them. You can't really use these stations like a treadmill or cycle at a gym because (as people who use them will attest to) you can't work and 'work-out' at the same time really. Exercising is taxing on the brain. Even if you don't notice it at the time, any type of multi-tasking puts a burden on your brain and is less effective per task than doing one thing at a time. So you will be exercising a little when using your computer or reading whilst walking on a treadmill but your focus will be reduced, potentially damaging the quality of your work. The loss in performance will depend on the type of work (Straker et al., 2009).

Walking to work is one area where some employers have tried to encourage behaviour change through some (albeit limited) walk to work interventions. These interventions and programmes have been dwarfed by cycle to work initiatives in the UK, which have been backed up by workplace bike incentive schemes and big investment in cycleways. Despite the fact that walking to work is great exercise (it is classed as moderately aerobic exercise at three miles an hour) and arguably safer and cheaper than cycling, walking still has not reached a critical mass for commuting purposes. I hope this changes, as walking to work brings the benefits to employers of a healthier and happier workforce and the opportunity to stamp their credibility as employers with corporate social responsibility and a belief in sustainability. I think that this will change when there is genuine support from the government for walking to work to run alongside employer-led programs which at the moment are half-hearted. Of course it is personal choice as to how people get to work and some employers may be concerned about being too interventionist if they encouraged walking more, but the same could be said about encouragement to use bikes.

It seems likely that employers will be more comfortable promoting active travel and employees less inclined to suspect their motives if the wider ethos of the workplace is that of a genuinely caring and supportive working environment. Promoting walking to work is one way that employers can show that they are supportive of their employees' health. Walking to work is likely to bring even greater benefits in terms of overall activity if it replicates the effect of walking to school, where studies have found that the morning walk to school is associated with higher overall moderate to vigorous physical activity throughout the day compared with travelling by car, bus, or train (Alexander et al., 2005). So, walking in the morning may be a particularly useful way to boost your exercise at other times and perhaps even become more productive generally.

Once at work, lunchtime seems a natural time to have a work walk. It is usually the longest break in the working day and splits the day nicely. A local-to-me lunchtime walking initiative lasting sixteen weeks, involving people who were physically inactive led to plenty of positive changes such as people feeling less tired and more energetic. This held true whether people walked in the summer or winter, dispelling the myth that walking is only for sunny weather. Even better, the positive changes lasted for several months even after people stopped walking (although I would hope that, given the great way that people felt as a result of walking at lunchtime that they would want to carry on with the walking breaks). Another group of lunchtime walkers had a significant improvement (lowering) of blood pressure after a park walk and this was even more significant than having a relaxation session (Thøgersen-Ntoumani et al., 2014). Parks or green corridors are accessible for many people at work (including people working from home); these are ideal environments for workplace walking.

Walking at work carries benefits that extend beyond the actual walk because people use the walk as an opportunity to reinforce their identity as 'walkers' and people interested and invested in their own wellbeing. This self-identity, coupled with the opportunity to learn more about wellbeing at work as an addition to lunchtime (or other time) walking sessions means that workplace walking has an important motivational role for people in terms of both wellbeing and potentially work performance. Because our self-identity is motivated by other people, the fact that people on 'work walks' walk as a group is a good way to motivate each other towards a better lifestyle. Changing attitudes and behaviours towards health are just as important to maintaining wellbeing as doing programmes, if not more so, so reinforcing a walk with positive change in diet, for example, could further enhance wellbeing.

So, to summarise the points made about walking as it relates to work:

- Most of us spend a lot of time sitting down at work, with its associated health risks. Walking is an effective way of mitigating these risks at work. Walking is more effective than standing desks or exercise/work stations in improving general wellbeing.

- Divergent thinking is enhanced during walking and also for a period after walking. This generates creative ideas which can be put into practice to solve problems. Walking at a steady speed with few distractions can also potentially assist with more focused thinking and with better recall of information.

- Walking breaks during the day can help with essential 'recovery' from work stresses, resetting internal functions and recharging our internal batteries.

- Walking can be a good way of strengthening teams and enabling people to get to know each other at work.

- As more people work from home, walking sessions in the local community could reduce isolation and create a sense of belonging.

Huge changes are happening right now in terms of work: where we do it, how much of it we do and what it looks like. However, for most people work still means sitting at a desk and moving very little. As we look for ways to improve both our wellbeing and also our performance at work, walking seems to me to be the perfect solution for both.

It is not just creative thinking or focus that makes a difference at work. Whether at work or out of it, confidence and resilience are great attributes to have and you won't be surprised to hear that walking is a good way of boosting both. In the next section I'll look at how walking helps you to face challenges and keep going towards your goals.

Confidence, Challenge and Resilience

You only have to look at a baby's face after he or she has taken their first steps to see the confidence generating power of walking. At that moment, that baby can do anything. They have conquered the greatest challenge in their short repertoire of challenges.

Confidence is about having self-belief. It is not about having an unrealistic sense of entitlement. It is about being able to be realistic about your capabilities and feeling secure that you will be able to act to meet the challenges you face. Confidence is a great trait to have because it has an impact on other people, who are likely to view you with respect and feel comfortable around you if you radiate a sense of inner security. Interestingly, most of us are drawn to people who are confident, even if their confidence is testament to an over-inflated ego or actual narcissism.

Yet confidence can be easily lost when we have setbacks in our lives. We quite often blame ourselves rather than the situation and this leaves us worried about how other people will view us. Being isolated from other people also tends to reduce confidence because confidence is partly derived from the feedback of other people; the lockdown associated with Covid-19 created the potential for people to lose confidence in this way, although this was partly mitigated by using online communication. The repercussions of being low on confidence include avoiding doing things because of the fear of failure. It may even lead to a resignation that life will plod on as it has been for the foreseeable future and that we are powerless to change anything, even when this feeling is accompanied by a sense of profound disappointment with life.

Confidence is all about your emotions; it is really about being able to handle the emotional outcomes of what happens. The amount of confidence you have is not fixed, you can lose it and gain it, as we all know you can feel confident one minute and not confident the next: no-one is confident all the time. Inner confidence is gained by personally accomplishing goals; persuading yourself of your own competency. There are lots of ways in which people can improve their confidence using self-development techniques or by working with someone as a coach. I'm not going to focus on these here because I want to highlight the way that walking is a great tool for creating confidence and one that I use in my own life.

Walking is a useful way to generate confident ways of thinking. One of the main ways it does this is by allowing us to experience mastering a particular activity, such as the activity of completing a walk, no matter how humble and get to the end. The sense of achievement upon finishing gives an emotional boost which lifts your confidence. The knowledge that you can rely on yourself creates what is termed 'self-efficacy' which spurs you on to believe in yourself. This self-belief is what gives you confidence.

The other key confidence booster with walking is sharing a walk with other people. You don't even have to say anything to learn confidence boosting skills from people around you. Walking as part of a walking group means you can settle into talking with people at your own pace and conversation is not 'head-on' but side to side, a much more comfortable and less threatening way to talk with strangers. In the safety of the group you can test out opinions, ask questions and get feedback about issues and you can share information at your own pace.

Walking on your own can also raise your level of confidence. In a society where it seems we derive our self-worth from what we believe other people to think about us, we can, instead, 'do our own thing' by walking. This simple act of going it alone can reinforce the sense of being comfortable in your own skin. Take it from me that other people will also be impressed that you have the confidence to walk on your own given the environment of fear that has been generated around people doing almost anything independently — especially for women.

I believe that even everyday walking can be treated as a mini daily achievement and, as such, brings benefits in terms of confidence and resilience. The beauty of walking is that you can pace it yourself, so if you set yourself one goal for a walk on one day and another the next. The fact that you can go for a walk and everything about the walk is within your own control is something that I feel is an important contribution both to independence, responsibility and also to boosting your own confidence and self-reliance.

Whether you choose to walk on your own or with others, the benefits of walking in terms of strengthening general psychological health are there for the taking. Since confidence is an emotional state, being able to better manage one's emotions enhances confidence. Walking in a quiet, green environment such as a forest, helps you to manage emotions by instilling a calm reassurance that is hard to quantify but undoubtedly can give you a feeling of positivity and reassurance.

There is an area of walking that has grown in popularity over the last ten years: walking as a challenge. Tens of thousands of people every year put on their walking boots and trek along roads, across forests and deserts in order to accomplish their goals or to raise money for charity. A quick search online returned hundreds of thousands of results for 'charity walk' and included treks raising funds for charities in the field of cancer, mental health, heart disease and just about every other charitable cause under the sun. Charity walks allow people to walk securely, whilst also demonstrating that they support a cause, giving them a sense of belonging and justification. In my experience, charity walkers may sometimes primarily just want to go for an adventure walk and see walking for a charity as a convenient pre-packaged and acceptable way to do this. I have mixed feelings about the industry that has grown up around charity walking but I do see it as a great way to introduce people to walking as a personal challenge. If it raises money for causes that matter to the participants, that is a very motivating bonus.

The walking and trekking holiday industry is massive. Adventure travel is worth in excess of £450 million per year, which is projected to reach over a staggering £1.2 billion a year by 2026 (Covid-19 will affect this projection). Of course walking is only a part of this mega-sector but walking, at levels from the very local to the 'extreme', is now a very significant commercial industry. People of all ages, seem to want to have some adventure (with the security of knowing that trips are properly organised and led) and challenge themselves. There are a thousand different motivations for people to do something big and dramatic but for many people a key one is the urge to define a new part of their life journey or to prove to themselves that they are capable of achieving a personal goal. Walking is therefore an affirming action that signifies personal growth, or dedication to a cause. To me, it is no co-incidence that there is a spike in people taking up adventure tourism in middle-age, a time when many people want to re-imagine themselves and start new adventures.

You could say that life today is full of challenge. Megatrends like globalisation, climate crisis and technological change all entail a series of stresses. To overcome these stresses requires hardiness and 'grit' — perseverance and passion for long term goals. The type of challenges that we face are those linked to a profound lack of control of our lives: news from around the world that is always on the bleak or frustrating side; keeping on top of a very precarious job situation for many people or trying to deal with the hundreds of other changes that we face because of the general shift to a more online, less forgiving world. The old-school (and simpler) challenges that used to be part of our lives have changed. Online technology does the hard work for us for everything from putting on the heating to replacing what we want to say with easy to interpret emoticons. We no longer have to struggle with shopping at the supermarket as we can get it all delivered to our door but if we did have to get there we would probably drive and the navigation would be taken care of by Google maps. So we don't actually have to find our way anywhere, we just follow a line on a map or even just a voice. Children no longer run around and get up to all sorts in the great outdoors like they used to; they are very likely to be found in front of a screen and very unlikely to be found up a tree, running around a field or making a den in a forgotten area of the garden.

It does seem that life now can be devoid of the sort of challenges that make us able to cope and grow. Challenges lead to the opportunity to solve problems and gain resilience. Without challenges we become bored. Boredom happens at a deep level and can affect you even if you are 'doing something' — it is the quality of the activity and the level of stimulation or challenge that your brain picks up on. One should not underestimate the damage that boredom causes: without sufficient challenge in our lives we can easily start to suffer psychological problems that we may not realise are linked to us not doing anything that is stimulating enough.

You can see this phenomenon in animals pacing backwards and forwards in a cage in a zoo. In humans, problems like depression and anxiety can be linked to lack of challenge.

Some types of walking, particularly adventure walking with an element of navigation, provide challenge in terms of preparing for the walk, pacing oneself, considering difficult elements, nutrition, what to do when the walk starts to feel tough, and many other aspects. This gives us an opportunity to use our cognitive skills to overcome problems in order to 'survive' in primitive terms. This means that we have to process, store, retrieve and act upon information from the environment, in other words we have to use our cognitive skills. This need for 'survival challenge' is something that we share with other animals that use navigational, tool-making or co-operative social skills in order to procure their food.

Walking means that you negotiate issues like routes, obstacles, time pressures and interacting with other people you might meet. Leading a walk brings responsibility, decision-making and dealing with mini-dramas and mini-crises that occur en route. Planning a walk, particularly if it involves other elements such as camping or organising equipment means that you learn techniques like breaking a task down into component parts, budgeting and communicating progress; these learning experiences are transferable to other non-walking tasks.

It is the contribution that walking challenges make to problem-solving that perhaps makes walking such a good fit with team-work. However, you don't need to walk in a familiar group for it to benefit social skills. Walking with new people in a group helps you to gain confidence and, importantly, be exposed to opinions that differ from your own. This exposure takes people outside the 'bubble' that each of us tends to live in, building resilience and coping mechanisms for times when things happen that we don't agree with and have no control over. Walking with others helps us to appreciate and respect the fact that people have differing views.

You don't need to be trekking through remote jungle for a walk to contribute to boosting resilience. Any walk can do this. Take that walk you might do every week through a local park. You might not realise it but making it something you complete on a regular basis means that you have demonstrated commitment — an important part of resilience. If you go on to do the walk despite bad weather, or when you are a bit tired, your brain will register this as determination and triumph over adversity and add a little bit to your resilience quota.

A further issue that I feel adds to both challenge and resilience and is as yet not very explored is the idea of the familiar versus the unfamiliar. Walking is particularly useful in providing challenge and generating resilience because, as we walk through a known area there is a mix of familiar and 'safe' features that reassure us and unfamiliar aspects that we learn from. I feel that our minds use this mix of old and new information to better embed learning and deal with challenges with a safety-net of familiarity, allowing us to take a few more calculated risks.

As day to day challenge is reduced because of the replacement of many tasks with technology, I feel that resilience is gradually evaporating away. People seem less able to cope with issues and the shock of events moving in a direction that is unexpected or unwelcome sometimes appears too much for them to accept, let alone deal with. All of this leads to practical problems such as not being able to solve the issue at hand and psychological problems such as feeling powerless, guilty about not being able to cope and anxious about the repercussions. No amount of listening to positive psychology on its own will be able to replace intrinsic resilience.

Resilience is the ability to 'bounce back' in the face of adversity and depends on coping mechanisms. Fortunately, these are mechanisms that we can acquire and add to through experience. Resilience is a dynamic process where we recover from traumatic experiences, adapt to deal with significant adversity and learn from this (hopefully). Key to resilience is the ability to continue to function in difficult circumstances. Resilience is much more pragmatic that just coping, in that it incorporates both actively confronting a situation and using the experience to drive forward in the future.

Walking with an element of challenge — and this could be just completing a short walk — is an ideal way to improve resilience. This is because it incorporates many aspects that we need to be resilient, both physiological and emotional. Walking means that we have to move and move in different environments and conditions, to which we have to adapt. Because resilience improves with repeated brief exposure to experiences, regular frequent walking is even more effective in creating resilience. You can also use walking as a tool, whilst practicing other coping mechanisms such as cognitive behavioural therapy or neuro-linguistic programming. Walking is a way for people to locate their inner strengths, strengths such as perseverance and self-reliance, and find new ways to deploy them. By focusing on what you can do you are more likely to adopt a more positive attitude to life in general.

Walking can give you a so-called 'mastery orientation' the ability to work out solutions to how to do things better, rather than feeling helpless. Mastery is the 'I love a challenge' and 'mistakes are our friends' mentality. Goals are important; the best goals for resilience are not just about performance but also about the ability to learn and use skills in the future (the potential for growth). By continuing to walk you feel more confident in your own ability to perform in other contexts, a key element of resilience. Walking encourages you to adopt a growth mindset and feel that you can achieve goals over time by persisting and believing that you can learn more and do more. This 'mindset' benefit of walking is extremely exciting. Walking helps you to continue to put in the effort to develop and succeed (Dweck, 2007).

Confidence and resilience are separate but related qualities. You can be confident without being resilient and vice versa but the two often go together. Walking strengthens both confidence and resilience. It helps us feel more secure about ourselves, our abilities and our communication with other people *and* it instils the practical tolerance to keeping going and succeeding towards our goals. Walking is a good mechanism for this because it is such a flexible pastime: your walking can grow with you. So, if you are feeling a little unsure and want a low profile new interest consider this scenario: firstly, you take up walking on your own locally or with a friend. This start in walking means that you can now call yourself a 'walker' (or a hiker or rambler if that fits); this then gives you the confidence to join a group of walkers who walk further afield. You may find yourself chatting with your fellow walkers, just small talk really but you click with a couple of people and, hey presto, you've made a few friends. Having proved to yourself that you can stay the course you start being a bit more ambitious and choose a few hill walks from the calendar of walks the group puts forward. This then leads to you seeking out more ambitious treks and so on. You can easily see how walking is an activity that sustains a gradual (or more rapid) change in confidence and resilience.

Becoming a confident and resilient walker does not just mean you become a better walker. The benefits of feeling more confident and gaining the practical endurance of attitude that you gain from your walking exploits are transferable to other areas of your life. So, for example if you struggle with keeping your promises to yourself you can refer yourself back to the fact that you consistently complete walks that you have signed up to. If you find being on time a challenge, walking provides a platform to test your commitment to not keeping people waiting.

Besides these direct associations, your brain picks up skills from walking and uses them to bolster how you function generally. For example, any walk (apart from on a treadmill) makes you more spatially aware of your surroundings and more familiar with changes in your environment. These two factors can subconsciously lead to more confidence in other unfamiliar settings, such as when you start a new job. It is also my observation that getting to know an area by walking around it is the only real way to feel that you 'belong' somewhere. In a world where we are detached from our surroundings more and more, it is somehow comforting to be able to find your way around an area, relying just on one's own insight and knowledge. The more you walk, the more you associate the mere act of walking with being confident in a type of place, be this city streets, a park or the open space of the countryside.

In my view, walking, and the improved personal mobility it brings equates to a type of freedom: the freedom to take risks and be in control of your own life. People, even with limited mobility, can taste the freedom of a walk under their own control. You do not need a car to make your own decision to go your own way in a walk. Anyone who takes a deliberate walk has made a personal choice to do this and this can go on to exemplify other personal choice decisions and to underline the capacity for that person to do their own thing.

On the resilience side, people often say to me that they feel that if they have completed a more challenging walk, they can do other things that they may have felt were difficult in the past, for example, have difficult conversations, complete practical tasks or become proactive on issues that they have put off for some time.

There is another aspect to walking that has been suggested though different sections of this book: that of personal growth. This is the journey that we take to fulfil our own potential and involves both conscious decisions and unknown quantities. The incredible thing is that walking makes a massive but at the same time almost imperceptible contribution to personal growth. Despite its contribution to wellbeing, confidence and enjoyment it is still seen as 'just walking'. The simplicity and everydayness of walking mean that it is a way for young people to explore life and their surroundings without being cooped up inside. For adults walking can be an equally liberating experience, delivering self-esteem and a realisation that there's a lot to explore in life.

So in summary, we can say the following in regard to confidence, challenge, resilience and walking:

- Walking increases your confidence, helping you to assess what you can realistically achieve and helping you to believe that you can attain your goals. It is also about being able to handle situations emotionally. People are innately drawn to others who are confident. However, confidence can be easily lost when we have setbacks. Achieving walking goals can give you confidence by making you self-reliant.

- The changing nature of challenges means that we have more limited opportunities to challenge ourselves with simple achievements day to day. This reduces our ability to gain confidence and resilience. Walking can create an opportunity to create substitute challenges that enable us to grow in ability and confidence.

- Resilience is the ability to persevere in adverse situations. Repeated walking is an ideal way to gain resilience and the resilience gained can help you in other contexts. Ongoing and progressively more challenging walking.

- Walking makes you spacially confident and gives you a sense of belonging and freedom.

I've given you a whirlwind tour of the history, beauty and utility of walking. From the creative to the life-extending: walking is truly multi-purpose, humble and yet awe-inspiring.

I'll conclude At Walking Pace by going through some of the 'loose ends' of walking. Firstly, I'll think about the practical considerations of walking and reflect on the fascinating subject of music whilst you walk.

I'll finish by reflecting on how walking may stride into the future, assisted by social-media and apps and accelerated by Covid and climate change.

At Walking Pace

Some Walking Choices

What is the right way to walk? A very basic question and one that has many answers. In this section I'll discuss the very basics of getting yourself up and walking and some ideas for walking for particular purposes. This is not to say that you should stick rigidly to these suggestions — one of the great things about walking is that it is an activity that you can mould to your own taste and that you can adapt as your circumstances change. Nevertheless, there are some useful tips that you could start with.

If you are generally fit and well then building up your walking should be fine, but having a regular health review is recommended to check on the overall state of your health. If you have existing health conditions, or feel unwell, then it is important that you consult with your doctor before any lifestyle change that could have an impact on your health and this includes taking up walking. Start small and build up your walking; don't expect to go from couch potato to mountain climber in a day!

As you might expect, one of the main things that affects how comfortably you walk and therefore how motivated you will be to walk effectively, is your footwear. There are thousands of boots, shoes and trainers out there for you to choose from and it really is a case of matching footwear to purpose. Short walks of less than half a mile are probably fine to do in your regular flat shoes or trainers (no high heels though). For longer walks along paths and streets supportive trainers or walking shoes are a great choice as long as they are the right size (don't try and squeeze your foot into footwear that is too small) You want a shoe that bends easily through the ball of the foot but remains fairly firm. A low heel works best, which is why a running shoe with thick cushioning in the heel is not the best choice. If you have any postural, gait or foot issues such as plantar fasciitis it is best to consult a doctor or chiropodist for advice on footwear. For off-road and hill walking get some proper walking boots with good support, there are plenty of great walking boots out there, both leather and synthetic.

Your gait is the way that you walk. Gait is very individual to you, so individual that investigators are able to pinpoint suspects though their gait and gait can be used for biometric security. Gait is a product of your basic physiology: the way your bones, muscles and joints work together and the changes that occur because of things like injury, age and repeated actions such as sitting for long periods every day or stooping a lot because of looking at screens. Improving your gait is possible by stopping bad habits like sitting all day and by using orthotics. Stretching and specialist exercise to improve your posture is another way to make your gait better. You can visit a foot specialist or athletic store to find out if you have any gait issues.

The way that you walk affects your mood. Even if you are faking it, walking with your head up and walking in a brisk way with your arms swinging will make you feel more upbeat compared with shuffling along and looking at your feet (Snodgrass, Sara E.; And Others, 1986). This is similar to the other better known mood-lifter of working your face into a smile artificially which also tricks your brain into a more positive state. Use walking to improve your posture. Start to look up and notice things above your eye line; keep your shoulders back rather than hunched up and walk with a pace that is not a dawdle (although there are some times when you might want to use walking as a way to slow down, with a focus more on what is around you such as botanicals), even if you are taking a meditative walk it is better to walk at a steady and not too slow pace, as this keeps your body in the best metabolic balance.

There are various theories on whether to walk on an empty stomach, have a snack before walking, or even walk after a big meal. This is really a case of whatever works for you. If you are going out for a session of speed-walking then maybe don't have an enormous feast but walking after a small meal is fine for most people. Recent studies have shown that it is a myth that you can't eat before exercising; in fact walking after a meal has been shown to be potentially beneficial in terms of lowering triglycerides which could help reduce the risk of heart problems. In addition, walking just after a meal seems to be more effective for weight loss than waiting for one hour to walk after a meal (Hijikata, 2011).

Walking when you are hungry is therefore not recommended. I do know of people who think they are furthering their weight loss ambitions by walking for long distances having eaten next to nothing; believe me this is counter-productive as you are likely to just eat more when you finish the walk. Indeed it can be risky to exercise if you have low blood sugar as this can leave you feeling dizzy and you won't enjoy the walk as you may spend the entire time feeling hungry. To mitigate against the risk of hunger ruining your walk I suggest taking some good, blood-sugar friendly snacks along such as fruit and nuts, or a flapjack or (my personal favourite) Bombay mix. Taking plenty of water along is important too if you are going for a fair old stretch. Stopping at a pub after a walk is great if you are walking with friends but keep alcohol consumption low for the sake of your general health.

Some people like to walk alone, some people like to walk with a couple of friends or with a group of walkers (perhaps joining local walking groups such as the Ramblers in the UK). There is no right or wrong way of walking. Solitary walking can be reflective and meditative or it can be driven and purposeful, either way it is a way to focus and rely on yourself. Walking on your own brings tremendous benefits in terms of building resilience and personal psychological strength. When walking on your own there is no pressure to talk with other people, leaving your mind free to wander and enter a creativity-friendly and recuperative state. Lone walking is also where you can become a true adventurer: venturing into new environments and perhaps, even using your walks as a metaphor for changes you will make in your life.

By contrast, group walking enables you to facilitate your dynamic social skills and gain support, feedback and motivation from other like-minded people. Walking in a group allows us to appreciate that everyone holds different opinions and that we can have a constructive relationship with people we may not necessarily agree with. Giving a commitment to walk with other people (if only to yourself) is a very powerful way of maintaining this simple lifestyle change and hopefully, once part of your life, you won't need any further encouragement to work walking into your life. Given time, you will be finding excuses to go walking.

A technique that I feel is particularly exciting is walking to music. Music has long been known to affect the brain in a positive way. Music has been a part of human culture since the beginning of humanity (just like walking) and has been proved to reduce stress, pain and the symptoms of depression. More than this, it also has a real impact on our abilities as playing and even listening to music help us to think, to perform tasks that need dexterity and help us to learn more effectively. Music even helps our brains to make more neurons which is why some people with diseases such as Alzheimer's and Parkinson's respond well to music. Even when people can't respond to other forms of stimulation, or verbally express themselves, their eyes light up when they hear music that they remember from the past. The type of music that you respond to best seems to depend on your personal background; any music can reach into your soul because memories associated with music are emotional memories, which never fade. Music has a profound effect on our emotions and we can interpret situations as being more positive or negative according to the mood of the music we listen to. However, it is perfectly possible to enjoy listen to sad songs without feeling down, or, indeed, feel sad listening to a catchy pop tune if we associate it with a negative experience.

What matters more as far as walking goes is tempo and volume. Playing music with an upbeat tempo (about 120-130 beats per minute) encourages us to walk to the beat of the music, more so than even walking to a metronome. We tend to synchronise our walking to the music. Moreover, we walk with more energy and vigour to music than without it. Walking to music motivates us to walk as we subconsciously challenge ourselves to keep in tempo with the beat (although this only works for music up to 145 beats per minute, beyond this we lose our motivation to walk because we feel overloaded). People also feel less tired during a walk when listening to music. Once again this is a trick of the brain: because we are using mental energy to listen to music this distracts us from feeling fatigued (or even in pain) and competes for our brain's attention, allowing us to walk for longer without feeling tired. This is also why music has a place in sports training and rehabilitation (Jabr, 2013).

As you may expect, adding music to walking can make you more creative, however this is not because music is a creative medium in itself. Yet again it comes down to the way the brain works. When you listen to music at a moderate volume your mind is working harder and this apparently triggers more abstract, creative thinking, once the music gets too loud however, it becomes distracting and creativity drops down (Mehta et al., 2012).

Of course, everyone is different and some people like to walk in silence, others with noise-cancelling headphones and others with some music going on around them but not enough to drown out other input like conversation or the sounds of the countryside. It is a matter of personal preference and perhaps even a generational thing: people, (like me) who grew up without the brain-filling quality of sound many headphones give you now might prefer to hear the 'real world' alongside music, whereas younger people might feel more comfortable immersing themselves in music as they walk. For safety reasons however, it is best to walk without blocking out all other sound, so wearing just one earpiece or listening to music from your device's own speaker rather than headphones is safest.

I know that it is unlikely that you will be walking as a group and all listening to the same music around you but if you were it would probably be an enjoyable and bonding experience. Beat-synchronised walking to music in a group makes us feel that we all have something in common in terms of our identity, indeed music in general has this effect which is why dancing has always been universally popular the world over. This phenomenon, known as 'muscular bonding' (moving together in synchrony), can be observed in marching bands and shows the role of the body as a mediator between the sonic properties of music (tempo, loudness) and physical experience.

Music then is a motivating force that fits perfectly with walking. I believe that walking and music both tap into very basic primitive instincts in our minds that are close to the heart of being a human being. I feel that walks with musical input are an under-used tool for general wellbeing.

Should you walk in the rain? This is very relevant question for anyone that lives in the United Kingdom, as I do. Honestly, most people don't want to walk in the rain. Of course, don't walk if it is dangerous to do so, be prepared for harsh conditions with the right clothing and footwear and always make sure you have the means to let others know if you are in difficulty on a walk. However, if you do end up being caught in pouring rain that soaks you literally to the skin whilst walking in Wales or the Lake District I bet you will remember this as one of the greatest walk adventures you had. If you are walking with other people in bad weather, my experience is that people keep each other going through the wind and rain and share great stories of the triumph of walking through the elements when they have dried off. These memories can last a lifetime.

The Future for Walking

So, what of the future? One thing is for sure, walking will be a greater part of it. The combination of national programmes encouraging walking and even prioritising pedestrians over other road users should both nudge people towards and enable them to feel more confident about walking. In the UK, for example, the Ramblers 'Walking for Health' initiative, supported by the National Lottery and Sport England has been running for almost two decades and involves volunteer walk leaders organising walks in their neighbourhood. The volunteers are trained to not only organise and lead the walks competently but also to encourage and support people with their walking. This scheme, aimed at the least active in society has reached many tens of thousands of walkers and has improved the physical and mental health of people up and down the UK. Thousands of weekly walks are advertised via the Walking for Health website and many have credited the programme with helping them to make new friends and reduce social isolation as well as improve their health and wellbeing.

'Walking for Health' has also shown the way in another way: the use of social media advertising to promote its walks as part of a 'digital-led behaviour change journey. Specifically, between June 2018 and June 2019 London Sport tried out Facebook advertising supported by text message, email and Facebook Messenger to support people to participate in Walking for Health walks. The London boroughs that were part of the Facebook pilot reported high conversion rates to actually joining local walking groups by people registering on the site. In comparison to more traditional ways of reaching out to people (posters and leaflets) the approach used in the pilot was cheaper to deliver per person and led to similar changes in activity levels. The pilot also succeeded in attracting a high proportion (71%) of people in the target group of 'less active' people (i.e. not meeting the Chief Medical Officer guidelines of 150 minutes activity per week).

Ironically, considering that walking is a way to moderate your screen-time by refocusing your time on living in the 'real world', using social media, whether it is Facebook, Meetup, Whatsapp or other social media platforms will inevitably be the best way to attract people to walking and keep people engaged in future. There are also mapping apps such as Viewranger, where walkers can share their walks and try routes generated by others. Of course you can also just go old-school and devise your own walking regime using local knowledge or maps.

The use of fitness and activity apps such as MapmyWalk, Walkmeter, Endomondo and Fitbit has rocketed in recent years and shows no signs of slowing its exponential growth. I have previously been a little sceptical of relying on apps and have sometimes been a little frustrated by people who constantly refer to them during a walk, or, even worse, inform everyone of key stats every half-kilometre or so. However, most people (thankfully) don't use apps in this way and my attitude has shifted to accept and even embrace the role of apps in walking. In order to back up my change of stance I looked into the research on whether fitness apps do encourage people to get walking and, importantly keep people walking. The results were very positive.

Stand-alone pedometers predated mobile apps and were all the rage during the '10,000 step challenge' heyday of 2010-2015. Follow-up studies of people who had taken part in pedometer challenges showed that participating in these challenges did, indeed, lead to greater levels of physical activity several years later (Harris et al., 2018). By introducing it to people, this basic technology put walking 'on the radar' and, it seems that plenty of people kept it on their radar and continued to include walking as part of their lifestyle as a result.

Smartphone apps, of course, make the humble pedometer look like something from a museum. Apps now measure distance walked, route followed, incline, theoretical calories burnt and a range of other metrics. They also add the dimension of an online global community and gamification to walking and other fitness activities. There are two main ways that activity apps may improve the take up and maintenance of walking: self-monitoring and social competition with others. By enabling people to keep a track on their walking, users can accurately know how far they have walked and how fast. As people can have a tendency to exaggerate their activity in their own minds, this reality check can be helpful in reaching personal goals. It can also be very motivating to feel that you are making progress along a particular walk.

However, it is the social and especially the gamification element of many apps that is likely to have the greatest impact on walking. By joining an app community, users become part of an often global cohort of users. This in itself creates a sense of belonging to a 'tribe' and encourages the aspiration to live up to the identity of that tribe, in this case active people, more specifically, walkers. This coupled with identifying yourself as belonging to this 'tribe' on the app or on other social media where you can share your personal achievement statistics and examples, creates a powerful incentive to engage. Competing against or comparing your activity with other app users is very motivational. In fact one study that analysed nearly 2,500 physical activity competitions and captured more than 800,000 person days of activity tracking over a period of a year, found that that during walking competitions the average user increases physical activity by 23%. This improvement was consistent for men and women; in fact where there was an equal mix of men and women activity levels increased the most; however when participants were very unevenly matched by ability then improvements dropped significantly (Shameli et al., 2017).

Overall then, walking activity apps do help people become interested in walking, monitor their own walking, compare it to other people's walking and take part in gamified challenges. The better the design of an app in terms of user-friendliness, real-time feedback, individualized elements and the provision of detailed information, the more beneficial it is likely to be. Obviously when gamification or social sharing is involved, the popularity of an app is a big factor in its take-up, level of activity and potential to have a long-term effect on walking.

So, a big shiny tick and gold star for walking activity apps. Or is it? By redefining walking as a 'biomedical' activity rather than as an activity that we all do as a matter of routine, apps can 'medicalise' walking as specifically concerned with wellbeing for a subset of the population (to the exclusion of its rather less sexy role as a means of transport) and categorise people into different good and bad groups — part of a bigger redefinition of people according to identity. Framing walking as being an extraordinary and rather middle-class activity runs the risk of further excluding some groups and reinforcing social divisions (S. Carter et al., 2018). This potential 'gentrification' of walking however is contradicted by the number of diverse groups of new walkers prompted by the Covid-19 pandemic. Walkers who took to the roads and tracks in this period were of all social strata, ethnic backgrounds and ages. Some digitally-mediated services aim to reduce social divisions and even use the potential of walking to help generate ideas to solve societal problems. Applications such as Meetup enable people of all backgrounds to meet and walk by registering themselves as part of a local group. The function of walking as a catalyst of social capital has always been around and has the potential to grow using digital technology. Indeed, the greater the perceived social value of a walking activity app, the more likely it is that people will use it over the long-term. Local authorities in the UK are funding walking projects in local parks with the aim of boosting public health.

The future will also potentially see a global change in priorities for road users. After a century of car domination, other road-users will likely gain precedence in many countries. The hierarchy of road users will ensure that those road users who can do the greatest harm have the greatest responsibility to reduce the danger or threat they may pose to others. For example, the Highway Code in the UK now gives pedestrians (as the most 'vulnerable' road users) priority in many road use situations, such as when crossing. Cars may also be stopped from partially parking on the pavement, which currently causes a hazard for vulnerable pedestrians. Many urban areas will accelerate plans to pedestrianise shopping and leisure streets, install walker-friendly street furniture such as benches and possibly even commission more public toilets.

New housing developments and workplaces are being designed with walking in mind. Improved lighting and wider pavements connecting places that people need and want to go to herald a new era where walking is seen as a normal rather than an extraordinary way to get from A to B. Employers may even start to routinely factor in work-time that includes walking around for periods of the day. I look forward to seeing all of these changes take shape.

There will be other future twists and turns along the road of walking. One thing is for sure: the future of walking will never stand still.

Conclusion

I have written this book perhaps as a reaction to the peculiar set of circumstances the world encountered in 2020 because of Covid-19. The uncertainty caused by the virus has led many people to walk more and others to be wary of walking. Undoubtedly, however, many people who have walked very little in the past now have a taste of life at walking speed and I hope that this sets a trend for the future.

This book is not a political commentary; I want people to practically grow to like and possibly even to love walking — not feel obliged to walk because of peer or political pressure. People make their own informed choices about life and how to live it. That said, there is plenty that recommends walking as part of the solution to sticky issues that are concerning people about the future. Walking is an important alternative means of travel during a period of increased awareness of the impact of motorised transport on our climate, as well as our health. I won't go into this in much detail as there is a wealth of informative literature out there for people to read. The Covid-19 pandemic has resulted in temporary measures to boost walking in cities in the UK becoming more permanent. This includes roads being closed to vehicles in residential and shopping areas. Some people welcome these moves; others are deeply hostile to them. At a local level this has led to a type of 'culture wars' scenario. I feel that suddenly imposing change when it alienates people is not wise. It is far better to win people over by enabling them to experience the wonder of walking: the purpose of this book.

This is homage to the ways that walking can lift your life. I am not a great explorer in the conventional sense, however walking has given me the freedom to be an explorer and adventurer every day; it is this accessibility and the humbleness of walking that I love so much and have shared in this short book.

Walking is a wonder: an activity that defined humanity itself and propelled mankind into roaming the planet and establishing civilisations. Despite this, most of us have rather taken walking for granted and as we put one foot in front of the other we mainly leave it at that, relying on this trusty action day after day and not thinking much about it. However, as I have articulated, there is just so much to walking. Our walking ancestors reach across to us from the past to give us clues about how they lived, moved and thought. Artists, writers, inventors and business people walked instinctively to help them relax, develop ideas and just because they felt like it. Alongside this, regular people also walked — because they had to, yes — but also to socialise and ponder.

Over the past hundred years or so the walking landscape has changed. Whereas prior to this, walking was the main mode of transport for the majority of people on the planet, the development of motorised transport rapidly relegated walking to an activity to be aspired away from. Work was transformed from the manual and active to the technology-driven and sedentary. Outside work, people needed to walk less and less. Walking became a 'time-waster' or even downright 'odd'. And yet, groups of people, the nature-loving ramblers, the quiet contemplators and the hard-core hill-walkers, all continued to keep walking as a leisure pursuit alive. Walking never went away, it may have lost its mojo for a while but its hard-core supporters did not care if it was untrendy or even ridiculed at times.

As technology has progressed, a parallel realisation has been made: our new lifestyles are not always good for us. So, the more sitting and less walking that we do the bigger, more unfit and more stressed we seem to become. The technological revolution of the first two decades or so of the 21st Century did much to further reduce our walking as activity needed for daily tasks has reached a new low and more and more of our leisure time is spent in front of a screen.

Very recently, however, things have been changing. People around the planet have noticed that life is better when walked. We have discovered that walking brings solid benefits to health and wellbeing and that walking in green space is therapeutic. Walking can be a tool to melt away the pounds, strengthen your heart or help you deal with anxiety. Walking can potentially help us to stave off dementia and keep us healthy in our old age. All you need to start is a pair of walking shoes and a route out of your front door.

Walking brings yet more benefits. Throughout history walking has been a creativity inspirer and aid to thinking. The power of walking has fuelled great writers and great artists. Who knows how many businesses have been born partly out of the inspiration that walking has provided? Walking brings people together and helps us to understand and respect each other, in the age of identity politics and confirmation bias. In a post-Covid-19, climatically compromised world we have never before needed walking as much as we do today because of its ability to change our lives for the better.

The zeitgeist moment for walking has arrived.

Conclusion

At Walking Pace

Appendix

Let me finish this book with some simple and short practical suggestions for walking for different purposes. Walking is the ultimate all-purpose exercise and endeavour and it may help to break down some of the key ways in which you could work it into your life.

Walking for fitness and weight control

Warming up: If you are walking for more than twenty minutes at a time, it is a good idea to warm up for thirty seconds or so using techniques like ankle circles (6-8 each direction, each foot), leg swings front and back 1 foot off the floor (15-20 each leg), pelvic loops (10 in each direction). There are plenty of suggestions online.

Posture: Keep your shoulders back and your abs tucked in. Look ahead and not down at your feet.

Stride: Walk at a natural stride, this will increase and you get fitter. Swing your arms naturally and not too aggressively.

Momentum: Walking involves landing each step on the heel with the foot in front of the body. Your weight then moves forward and you push off from the toes of that foot. The stronger the 'roll' of your foot, the more power you will have.

Distance/Time: For absolute beginners to walking focus on walking for thirty minutes, spread through the day and then increasing the time you spend walking. Instead of distance to start with, think more of trips 'round the block' in an urban environment. Once you have got into the habit of walking you can then start increasing your pace/distance walked/time walked.

Walking for mental wellbeing

In addition to the points made in the previous section:

Location: walking in a forest can be really helpful to the way that you feel. In addition, green spaces in general and places near water (riversides, near lakes, beaches and even canals) are restful and may be considered therapeutic places to walk.

Mindful walking: Being mindful of your internal state (your senses, breathing and movement of your limbs) as well as noticing the environment around you, whilst clearing your mind of past and future issues.

Speed: Walk at a steady pace, whatever is right for you. Your natural walking pace should, as you get fitter, increase. Don't feel compelled to continuously walk; stop to look around if you feel like it.

Company: Walking with other people gives a feeling of security and togetherness and helps you to practice and strengthen your social skills.

Walking for thinking and work

Ideas and Creativity: Walking at a steady pace in any surroundings whilst letting your mind 'wander' is good for the generation of creative ideas. The capacity to generate these ideas carries in for some time after you stop walking, so a post-walk brainstorm sounds ideal.

Walking for thinking: Some people find walking at a speed of about three miles an hour helpful for solving problems. Actively thinking whilst walking means more work for the brain, since walking does draw on your mental energy, so other distractions should be kept to a minimum.

Walking for work recuperation: Getting to work on foot and/or having walking breaks can break up the day and allow your mind to rest and recuperate. Even if you work from home, this can be helpful to recharging your batteries.

A walking break from work should not mean thinking about your work as you walk; rather it should mean clearing you mind and soaking in your surroundings.

Location: Any walking is good, but walking in green spaces is the most likely to have a positive impact on your wellbeing.

Walking for challenge

Any walk can be a challenge walk. Turn each walk into a mini-adventure by seeing what is different around you, or taking pleasure in what is the same.

You can challenge yourself to walk just a bit further, for a little longer, or to walk in a more hilly or unexplored environment.

Walking can use other skills, like planning and navigation. Put these skills to the test.

You can use walking as a metaphor for other areas of your life and be spurred on to make positive changes by accomplishing your walking goals.

Appendix

At Walking Pace

At Walking Pace

Bibliography

Alexander, L. M., Inchley, J., Todd, J., Currie, D., Cooper, A. R., & Currie, C. (2005). The broader impact of walking to school among adolescents: seven day accelerometry based study. BMJ, 331(7524), 1061–1062.
https://doi.org/10.1136/bmj.38567.382731.ae

Al-Yahya, E., Dawes, H., Smith, L., Dennis, A., Howells, K., & Cockburn, J. (2011). Cognitive motor interference while walking: A systematic review and meta-analysis. Neuroscience & Biobehavioral Reviews, 35(3), 715–728.
https://doi.org/10.1016/j.neubiorev.2010.08.008

Audrey, S., & Procter, S. (2015). Employers' views of promoting walking to work: a qualitative study. *International Journal of Behavioral Nutrition and Physical Activity, 12*(1), 0.
https://doi.org/10.1186/s12966-015-0174-8

Baker, G., Gray, S. R., Wright, A., Fitzsimons, C., Nimmo, M., Lowry, R., & Mutrie, N. (2008). The effect of a pedometer-based community walking intervention 'Walking for Wellbeing in the West' on physical activity levels and health outcomes: a 12-week randomized controlled trial. *International Journal of Behavioral Nutrition and Physical Activity, 5*(1), 44. https://doi.org/10.1186/1479-5868-5-44

Baker, R., Coenen, P., Howie, E., Lee, J., Williamson, A., & Straker, L. (2018). A detailed description of the short-term musculoskeletal and cognitive effects of prolonged standing for office computer work. *Ergonomics, 61*(7), 877–890. https://doi.org/10.1080/00140139.2017.1420825

Bang, K.-S., Lee, I., Kim, S., Lim, C. S., Joh, H.-K., Park, B.-J., & Song, M. K. (2017). The Effects of a Campus Forest-Walking Program on Undergraduate and Graduate Students' Physical and Psychological Health. *International Journal of Environmental Research and Public Health, 14*(7), 728. https://doi.org/10.3390/ijerph14070728

Bemben, M. G., Clary, S. R., Barnes, C., Bemben, D.
A., & Knehans, A. W. (2006). Effects of Ballates, Step
Aerobics, and Walking on Balance in Women Aged
50 to 75 Years. *Medicine & Science in Sports &
Exercise*, *38*(Supplement), S445.
https://doi.org/10.1249/00005768-200605001-
02744

Bonato, M., Bossolasco, S., Galli, L., Pavei, G., Testa,
M., Bertocchi, C., Galvano, E., Balconi, G., Lazzarin,
A., Merati, G., La Torre, A., & Cinque, P. (2012).
Moderate aerobic exercise (brisk walking) increases
bone density in cART-treated persons. *Journal of the
International AIDS Society*, *15*(6(Suppl 4)), 0.
https://doi.org/10.7448/ias.15.6.18318

Campbell, J. P., & Turner, J. E. (2018). Debunking
the Myth of Exercise-Induced Immune Suppression:
Redefining the Impact of Exercise on Immunological
Health Across the Lifespan. *Frontiers in
Immunology*, *9*, 0.
https://doi.org/10.3389/fimmu.2018.00648

Carter, S. E., Draijer, R., Holder, S. M., Brown, L.,
Thijssen, D. H. J., & Hopkins, N. D. (2018). Regular
walking breaks prevent the decline in cerebral blood

flow associated with prolonged sitting. *Journal of Applied Physiology, 125*(3), 790–798. https://doi.org/10.1152/japplphysiol.00310.2018

Cavalcante, B. R., Germano-Soares, A. H., Gerage, A. M., Leicht, A., Tassitano, R. M., Bortolotti, H., de Mello Franco, F. G., Wolosker, N., Cucato, G. G., & Ritti-Dias, R. M. (2018). Association between physical activity and walking capacity with cognitive function in peripheral artery disease patients. European Journal of Vascular and Endovascular Surgery, 55(5), 672–678. https://doi.org/10.1016/j.ejvs.2018.02.010

Carter, S., Green, J., & Speed, E. (2018). Digital technologies and the biomedicalisation of everyday activities: The case of walking and cycling. Sociology Compass, 12(4), e12572. https://doi.org/10.1111/soc4.12572

CDC. Adult Overweight and Obesity | Overweight & Obesity (2020). CDC. https://www.cdc.gov/obesity/adult/index.html

Crone, D. (2007). Walking back to health: A qualitative investigation into service users' experiences of a walking project. *Issues in Mental Health Nursing*, *28*(2), 167–183. https://doi.org/10.1080/01612840601096453

Crust, L., Keegan, R., Piggott, D., & Swann, C. (2011). Walking the Walk: A Phenomenological Study of Long Distance Walking. *Journal of Applied Sport Psychology*, *23*(3), 243–262. https://doi.org/10.1080/10413200.2010.548848

Cycling and Walking 'on prescription' in the West Midlands. (2020). West Midlands Combined Authority. https://www.wmca.org.uk/news/cycling-and-walking-on-prescription-in-the-west-midlands/

de Bloom, J., Kinnunen, U., & Korpela, K. (2014). Exposure to nature versus relaxation during lunch breaks and recovery from work: development and design of an intervention study to improve workers' health, well-being, work performance and creativity. *BMC Public Health*, *14*(1), 0. https://doi.org/10.1186/1471-2458-14-488

de Bloom, J., Sianoja, M., Korpela, K., Tuomisto, M., Lilja, A., Geurts, S., & Kinnunen, U. (2017). Effects of park walks and relaxation exercises during lunch breaks on recovery from job stress: Two randomized controlled trials. *Journal of Environmental Psychology*, *51*, 14–30. https://doi.org/10.1016/j.jenvp.2017.03.006

de Moura, B. P., Marins, J. C. B., & Amorim, P. R. S. (2011). Self selected walking speed in overweight adults: Is this intensity enough to promote health benefits? *Apunts. Medicina de l'Esport*, *46*(169), 11–15. https://doi.org/10.1016/j.apunts.2010.10.004

Dempsey, P. C., Larsen, R. N., Sethi, P., Sacre, J. W., Straznicky, N. E., Cohen, N. D., Cerin, E., Lambert, G. W., Owen, N., Kingwell, B. A., & Dunstan, D. W. (2016). Benefits for Type 2 Diabetes of Interrupting Prolonged Sitting With Brief Bouts of Light Walking or Simple Resistance Activities. *Diabetes Care*, *39*(6), 964–972. https://doi.org/10.2337/dc15-2336

Diehr, P., & Hirsch, C. (2010). Health Benefits of Increased Walking for Sedentary, Generally Healthy Older Adults: Using Longitudinal Data to Approximate an Intervention Trial. *The Journals of Gerontology Series A: Biological Sciences and Medical Sciences*, *65A*(9), 982–989. https://doi.org/10.1093/gerona/glq070

Duvall, J. (2011). Enhancing the benefits of outdoor walking with cognitive engagement strategies. *Journal of Environmental Psychology, 31*(1), 27–35. https://doi.org/10.1016/j.jenvp.2010.09.003

Duvivier, B. M. F. M. (2020, August 31). *Benefits of Substituting Sitting with Standing and Walking in Free-Living Conditions for Cardiometabolic Risk Markers, Cognition and Mood in Overweight Adults.* Frontiers. https://www.frontiersin.org/articles/10.3389/fphys.2017.00353/full

Dweck, C. S. (2007). *Mindset: The New Psychology of Success* (Illustrated ed.). Ballantine Books.

Edensor, T. (2010). Walking in rhythms: place, regulation, style and the flow of experience. *Visual Studies, 25*(1), 69–79. https://doi.org/10.1080/14725861003606902

Freeman, E., Akhurst, J., Bannigan, K., & James, H. (2016). Benefits of walking and solo experiences in UK wild places. *Health Promotion International,* daw036. https://doi.org/10.1093/heapro/daw036

Frydenberg, E. (2017). *Coping and the Challenge of Resilience* (1st ed. 2017 ed.). Palgrave Macmillan.

Gába, A., Cuberek, R., Svoboda, Z., Chmelík, F., Pelclová, J., Lehnert, M., & Frömel, K. (2016). The effect of brisk walking on postural stability, bone mineral density, body weight and composition in women over 50 years with a sedentary occupation: a randomized controlled trial. *BMC Women's Health, 16*(1), 0. https://doi.org/10.1186/s12905-016-0343-1

Gidlow, C. J., Jones, M. V., Hurst, G., Masterson, D., Clark-Carter, D., Tarvainen, M. P., Smith, G., & Nieuwenhuijsen, M. (2016). Where to put your best foot forward: Psycho-physiological responses to walking in natural and urban environments. *Journal of Environmental Psychology, 45*, 22–29. https://doi.org/10.1016/j.jenvp.2015.11.003

Gilson, N. D., Puig-Ribera, A., McKenna, J., Brown, W. J., Burton, N. W., & Cooke, C. B. (2009). Do walking strategies to increase physical activity reduce reported sitting in workplaces: a randomized control trial. *International Journal of Behavioral Nutrition and Physical Activity, 6*(1), 43. https://doi.org/10.1186/1479-5868-6-43

Gordon-Larsen, P., Hou, N., Sidney, S., Sternfeld, B., Lewis, C. E., Jacobs, D. R., & Popkin, B. M. (2008). Fifteen-year longitudinal trends in walking patterns and their impact on weight change. *The American Journal of Clinical Nutrition, 89*(1), 19–26. https://doi.org/10.3945/ajcn.2008.26147

Gros, F., Harper, C., & Howe, J. (2015). *A Philosophy of Walking* (Reprint ed.). Verso.

Hackett, R. A., Davies-Kershaw, H., Cadar, D., Orrell, M., & Steptoe, A. (2018). Walking Speed, Cognitive Function, and Dementia Risk in the English Longitudinal Study of Ageing. Journal of the American Geriatrics Society, 66(9), 1670–1675. https://doi.org/10.1111/jgs.15312

Harris, T., Kerry, S. M., Limb, E. S., Furness, C., Wahlich, C., Victor, C. R., Iliffe, S., Whincup, P. H., Ussher, M., Ekelund, U., Fox-Rushby, J., Ibison, J., DeWilde, S., McKay, C., & Cook, D. G. (2018). Physical activity levels in adults and older adults 3–4 years after pedometer-based walking interventions: Long-term follow-up of participants from two randomised controlled trials in UK primary care.

PLOS   Medicine,15(3),e1002526.
https://doi.org/10.1371/journal.pmed.1002526

Hennekens, C. (2000). Brisk walking and vigorous exercise provide similar cardiovascular disease benefits. *European Heart Journal, 21*(19), 1559. https://doi.org/10.1053/euhj.2000.2197

Hijikata, Y. (2011). Walking just after a meal seems to be more effective for weight loss than waiting for one hour to walk after a meal. *International Journal of General Medicine,* 447. https://doi.org/10.2147/ijgm.s18837

Hillman, C. H., Pontifex, M. B., Raine, L. B., Castelli, D. M., Hall, E. E., & Kramer, A. F. (2009). The effect of acute treadmill walking on cognitive control and academic achievement in preadolescent children. *Neuroscience, 159*(3), 1044–1054. https://doi.org/10.1016/j.neuroscience.2009.01.057

Ho, C.-F., Maa, S.-H., Shyu, Y.-I. L., Lai, Y.-T., Hung, T.-C., & Chen, H.-C. (2012). Effectiveness of Paced Walking to Music at Home for Patients with COPD. *COPD: Journal of Chronic Obstructive Pulmonary*

Disease, 9(5), 447–457.
https://doi.org/10.3109/15412555.2012.685664

Horton, J., Christensen, P., Kraftl, P., & Hadfield-
Hill, S. (2013). 'Walking … just walking': how
children and young people's everyday pedestrian
practices matter. *Social & Cultural Geography*, 15(1),
94–115.
https://doi.org/10.1080/14649365.2013.864782

H.S.E. (2020). *Should VDU users be given breaks?*
HSE.
https://www.hse.gov.uk/contact/faqs/vdubreaks.ht
m

Hui, S. S.-C., Xie, Y. J., Woo, J., & Kwok, T. C.-Y.
(2015). Effects of Tai Chi and Walking Exercises on
Weight Loss, Metabolic Syndrome Parameters, and
Bone Mineral Density: A Cluster Randomized
Controlled Trial. *Evidence-Based Complementary
and Alternative Medicine*, 2015, 1–10.
https://doi.org/10.1155/2015/976123

Jabr, F. (2013a, March 20). *Let's Get Physical: The
Psychology of Effective Workout Music*. Scientific
American.

https://www.scientificamerican.com/article/psychol
ogy-workout-music/

Jabr, F. (2013b, March 20). *Let's Get Physical: The Psychology of Effective Workout Music*. Scientific American.
https://www.scientificamerican.com/article/psychol
ogy-workout-music/

Jin, P. (1992). Efficacy of Tai Chi, brisk walking, meditation, and reading in reducing mental and emotional stress. *Journal of Psychosomatic Research*, *36*(4), 361–370.
https://doi.org/10.1016/0022-3999(92)90072-a

Johansson, M., Hartig, T., & Staats, H. (2011). Psychological Benefits of Walking: Moderation by Company and Outdoor Environment. *Applied Psychology: Health and Well-Being*, *3*(3), 261–280.
https://doi.org/10.1111/j.1758-0854.2011.01051.x

Kakanis, M., Peake, J., Hooper, S., Gray, B., & Marshall-Gradisnik, S. (2010). The open window of susceptibility to infection after acute exercise in healthy young male elite athletes. *Journal of Science*

and Medicine in Sport, 13, e85–e86.
https://doi.org/10.1016/j.jsams.2010.10.642

Keinänen, M. (2015). Taking your mind for a walk: a qualitative investigation of walking and thinking among nine Norwegian academics. *Higher Education, 71*(4), 593–605.
https://doi.org/10.1007/s10734-015-9926-2

Kelly, P., Williamson, C., Niven, A. G., Hunter, R., Mutrie, N., & Richards, J. (2018). Walking on sunshine: scoping review of the evidence for walking and mental health. *British Journal of Sports Medicine, 52*(12), 800–806.
https://doi.org/10.1136/bjsports-2017-098827

Kemoun, G., Thibaud, M., Roumagne, N., Carette, P., Albinet, C., Toussaint, L., Paccalin, M., & Dugué, B. (2010b). Effects of a Physical Training Programme on Cognitive Function and Walking Efficiency in Elderly Persons with Dementia. *Dementia and Geriatric Cognitive Disorders, 29*(2), 109–114.
https://doi.org/10.1159/000272435

Khamsi, R. (2007). *Walking on two feet was an energy-saving step.* New Scientist.

https://www.newscientist.com/article/dn12269-walking-on-two-feet-was-an-energy-saving-step/#:%7E:text=The%20study%2C%20which%20used%20treadmills,ancestors%20to%20take%20up%2obipedalism.

Kimura, F., Shimizu, K., Akama, T., Akimoto, T., Kuno, S., & Kono, I. (2006). The Effects of Walking Exercise Training on Immune Response in Elderly Subjects. *International Journal of Sport and Health Science, 4,* 508–514. https://doi.org/10.5432/ijshs.4.508

Kopp, M., Steinlechner, M., Ruedl, G., Ledochowski, L., Rumpold, G., & Taylor, A. H. (2012). Acute effects of brisk walking on affect and psychological well-being in individuals with type 2 diabetes. *Diabetes Research and Clinical Practice, 95*(1), 25–29. https://doi.org/10.1016/j.diabres.2011.09.017

Kume, S., Nishimura, Y., Mizuno, K., Sakimoto, N., Hori, H., Tamura, Y., Yamato, M., Mitsuhashi, R., Akiba, K., Koizumi, J., Watanabe, Y., & Kataoka, Y. (2017). Music Improves Subjective Feelings Leading to Cardiac Autonomic Nervous Modulation: A Pilot

Study. *Frontiers in Neuroscience, 11,* 0.
https://doi.org/10.3389/fnins.2017.00108

Kuo, C.-Y., & Yeh, Y.-Y. (2016). Sensorimotor-
Conceptual Integration in Free Walking Enhances
Divergent Thinking for Young and Older Adults.
Frontiers in Psychology, 7, 1.
https://doi.org/10.3389/fpsyg.2016.01580

Ledochowski, L., Ruedl, G., Taylor, A. H., & Kopp, M.
(2015). Acute Effects of Brisk Walking on Sugary
Snack Cravings in Overweight People, Affect and
Responses to a Manipulated Stress Situation and to a
Sugary Snack Cue: A Crossover Study. *PLOS ONE,*
10(3), e0119278.
https://doi.org/10.1371/journal.pone.0119278

Leisman, G., Moustafa, A., & Shafir, T. (2016).
Thinking, Walking, Talking: Integratory Motor and
Cognitive Brain Function. *Frontiers in Public Health,*
4, 0. https://doi.org/10.3389/fpubh.2016.00094

Leman, M., Moelants, D., Varewyck, M., Styns, F.,
van Noorden, L., & Martens, J.-P. (2013). Activating
and Relaxing Music Entrains the Speed of Beat

Synchronized Walking. *PLoS ONE, 8*(7), e67932.
https://doi.org/10.1371/journal.pone.0067932

Leon, A. S., Conrad, J., Hunninghake, D. B., &
Serfass, R. (1979). Effects of a vigorous walking
program on body composition, and carbohydrate and
lipid metabolism of obese young men. *The American
Journal of Clinical Nutrition, 32*(9), 1776–1787.
https://doi.org/10.1093/ajcn/32.9.1776

Lovejoy, C. O. (1988). Evolution of Human Walking.
Scientific American, 259(5), 118–125.
https://doi.org/10.1038/scientificamerican1188-118

Marselle, M., Irvine, K., & Warber, S. (2013). Walking
for Well-Being: Are Group Walks in Certain Types of
Natural Environments Better for Well-Being than
Group Walks in Urban Environments? *International
Journal of Environmental Research and Public
Health, 10*(11), 5603–5628.
https://doi.org/10.3390/ijerph10115603

Marselle, M., Warber, S., & Irvine, K. (2019).
Growing Resilience through Interaction with Nature:
Can Group Walks in Nature Buffer the Effects of
Stressful Life Events on Mental Health?

International Journal of Environmental Research and Public Health, 16(6), 986. https://doi.org/10.3390/ijerph16060986

Martyn-St James, M., & Carroll, S. (2008). Meta-analysis of walking for preservation of bone mineral density in postmenopausal women. *Bone, 43*(3), 521–531. https://doi.org/10.1016/j.bone.2008.05.012

Mehta, R., Zhu, R. J., & Cheema, A. (2012). Is Noise Always Bad? Exploring the Effects of Ambient Noise on Creative Cognition. *Journal of Consumer Research, 39*(4), 784–799. https://doi.org/10.1086/665048

Mobily, K. E., Rubenstein, L. M., Lemke, J. H., O'Hara, M. W., & Wallace, R. B. (1996). Walking and Depression in a Cohort of Older Adults: The Iowa 65+ Rural Health Study. *Journal of Aging and Physical Activity, 4*(2), 119–135. https://doi.org/10.1123/japa.4.2.119

Morgan, A. L., Tobar, D. A., & Snyder, L. (2010). Walking Toward a New Me: The Impact of Prescribed Walking 10,000 Steps/Day on Physical and Psychological Well-Being. *Journal of Physical*

Activity and Health, 7(3), 299–307.
https://doi.org/10.1123/jpah.7.3.299

Morita, E., Fukuda, S., Nagano, J., Hamajima, N.,
Yamamoto, H., Iwai, Y., Nakashima, T., Ohira, H., &
Shirakawa, T. (2007). Psychological effects of forest
environments on healthy adults: Shinrin-yoku
(forest-air bathing, walking) as a possible method of
stress reduction. *Public Health, 121*(1), 54–63.
https://doi.org/10.1016/j.puhe.2006.05.024

Morita, E., Imai, M., Okawa, M., Miyaura, T., &
Miyazaki, S. (2011). A before and after comparison of
the effects of forest walking on the sleep of a
community-based sample of people with sleep
complaints. *BioPsychoSocial Medicine, 5*(1), 13.
https://doi.org/10.1186/1751-0759-5-13

Morris, J. N., & Hardman, A. E. (1997). Walking to
Health. *Sports Medicine, 23*(5), 306–332.
https://doi.org/10.2165/00007256-199723050-
00004

Murphy, Marie., Neville, Alan., Neville, Charlotte.,
Biddle, Stuart., & Hardman, Adrianne. (2002).
Accumulating brisk walking for fitness,

cardiovascular risk, and psychological health. *Medicine & Science in Sports & Exercise, 34*(9), 1468–1474. https://doi.org/10.1097/00005768-200209000-00011

Murphy, M. H., Murtagh, E. M., Boreham, C. A. G., Hare, L. G., & Nevill, A. M. (2006). The effect of a worksite based walking programme on cardiovascular risk in previously sedentary civil servants [NCT00284479]. *BMC Public Health, 6*(1), 0. https://doi.org/10.1186/1471-2458-6-136

Nehlsen-Cannarella, Sandra, L., Nieman, David, C., Balk-Lamberton, Anne, J., Markoff, Patricia. A., Chritton, Douglas, B. W., Gusewitch, Gary., & Lee, Jerry, W. (1991). The effects of moderate exercise training on immune response. *Medicine & Science in Sports & Exercise, 23*(1), 64???70. https://doi.org/10.1249/00005768-199101000-00011

Nelson, M. E., & Folta, S. C. (2008). Further evidence for the benefits of walking. *The American Journal of Clinical Nutrition, 89*(1), 15–16. https://doi.org/10.3945/ajcn.2008.27118

New exhibit showcases importance of walking in Cree culture. (2016). CBC News. https://www.cbc.ca/news/canada/north/footprints-exhibit-walking-cree-culture-quebec-1.3753835

Nieman, D. C., & Pedersen, B. K. (1999). Exercise and Immune Function. *Sports Medicine, 27*(2), 73–80. https://doi.org/10.2165/00007256-199927020-00001

Oppezzo, M., & Schwartz, D. L. (2014). Give your ideas some legs: The positive effect of walking on creative thinking. *Journal of Experimental Psychology: Learning, Memory, and Cognition, 40*(4), 1142–1152. https://doi.org/10.1037/a0036577

Palmer, L. K. (1995). Effects of a Walking Program on Attributional Style, Depression, and Self-Esteem in Women. *Perceptual and Motor Skills, 81*(3), 891–898. https://doi.org/10.2466/pms.1995.81.3.891

Pasanen, T, White, M., Wheeler, B., Garrett, J., Elliott, L., Neigh*bourhood blue space, health and wellbeing: The mediating role of different types of physical activity. Environment International, Volume 131* *https://doi.org/10.1016/j.envint.2019.105016.*

Patterson, R., Frith, E., & Loprinzi, P. (2018). The Experimental Effects of Acute Walking on Cognitive Creativity Performance. *Journal of Behavioral Health, 0,* 113. https://doi.org/10.5455/jbh.20180415053930

Pedersen, B. K., & Hoffman-Goetz, L. (2000). Exercise and the Immune System: Regulation, Integration, and Adaptation. *Physiological Reviews, 80*(3), 1055–1081. https://doi.org/10.1152/physrev.2000.80.3.1055

Phillips, W. T., Kiernan, M., & King, A. C. (2003). Physical Activity as a Nonpharmacological Treatment for Depression: A Review. *Complementary Health Practice Review, 8*(2), 139–152. https://doi.org/10.1177/1076167502250792

Prang, T. C. (2019). The African ape-like foot of Ardipithecus ramidus and its implications for the origin of bipedalism. *ELife, 8,* 0. https://doi.org/10.7554/elife.44433

Priest, P. (2007). The Healing Balm Effect. *Journal of Health Psychology, 12*(1), 36–52. https://doi.org/10.1177/1359105307071734

Puig-Ribera, A., McKenna, J., Gilson, N., & Brown, W. J. (2008). Change in work day step counts, wellbeing and job performance in Catalan university employees: a randomised controlled trial. *Promotion & Education, 15*(4), 11–16. https://doi.org/10.1177/1025382308097693

Raichlen, D. A., Wood, B. M., Gordon, A. D., Mabulla, A. Z. P., Marlowe, F. W., & Pontzer, H. (2013). Evidence of Levy walk foraging patterns in human hunter-gatherers. *Proceedings of the National Academy of Sciences, 111*(2), 728–733. https://doi.org/10.1073/pnas.1318616111

Rasmussen, L. J. H., Caspi, A., Ambler, A., Broadbent, J. M., Cohen, H. J., d'Arbeloff, T., Elliott, M., Hancox, R. J., Harrington, H., Hogan, S., Houts, R., Ireland, D., Knodt, A. R., Meredith-Jones, K., Morey, M. C., Morrison, L., Poulton, R., Ramrakha, S., Richmond-Rakerd, L., ... Moffitt, T. E. (2019). Association of Neurocognitive and Physical Function With Gait Speed in Midlife. *JAMA Network Open, 2*(10), e1913123. https://doi.org/10.1001/jamanetworkopen.2019.13123

Richardson, C. R., Newton, T. L., Abraham, J. J., Sen, A., Jimbo, M., & Swartz, A. M. (2008). A Meta-Analysis of Pedometer-Based Walking Interventions and Weight Loss. *The Annals of Family Medicine*, 6(1), 69–77. https://doi.org/10.1370/afm.761

Robertson, R., Robertson, A., Jepson, R., & Maxwell, M. (2012). Walking for depression or depressive symptoms: A systematic review and meta-analysis. *Mental Health and Physical Activity*, 5(1), 66–75. https://doi.org/10.1016/j.mhpa.2012.03.002

Roe, J., & Aspinall, P. (2011). The restorative benefits of walking in urban and rural settings in adults with good and poor mental health. Health & Place, 17(1), 103–113. https://doi.org/10.1016/j.healthplace.2010.09.003

Sakuragi, S., & Sugiyama, Y. (2006). Effects of Daily Walking on Subjective Symptoms, Mood and Autonomic Nervous Function. Journal of Physiological Anthropology, 25(4), 281–289. https://doi.org/10.2114/jpa2.25.281

Shameli, A., Althoff, T., Saberi, A., & Leskovec, J. (2017). How Gamification Affects Physical Activity.

Proceedings of the 26th International Conference on World Wide Web Companion - WWW '17 Companion, 1. https://doi.org/10.1145/3041021.3054172

Sharma, A., Madaan, V., & Petty, F. D. (2006). Exercise for Mental Health. *The Primary Care Companion to The Journal of Clinical Psychiatry*, *08*(02), 106. https://doi.org/10.4088/pcc.v08n0208a

Shin, Y.-K., Kim, D. J., Jung-Choi, K., Son, Y., Koo, J.-W., Min, J.-A., & Chae, J.-H. (2013). Differences of psychological effects between meditative and athletic walking in a forest and gymnasium. *Scandinavian Journal of Forest Research*, *28*(1), 64–72. https://doi.org/10.1080/02827581.2012.706634

Snodgrass, Sara E.; And Others. (1986, August). *The Effects of Walking Behavior on Mood.* https://eric.ed.gov/?id=ED284086

Sockol, M. D., Raichlen, D. A., & Pontzer, H. (2007). Chimpanzee locomotor energetics and the origin of human bipedalism. *Proceedings of the National*

Academy of Sciences, *104*(30), 12265–12269.
https://doi.org/10.1073/pnas.0703267104

Song, C., Ikei, H., Park, B.-J., Lee, J., Kagawa, T., &
Miyazaki, Y. (2018). Psychological Benefits of
Walking through Forest Areas. *International Journal
of Environmental Research and Public Health*,
15(12), 2804.
https://doi.org/10.3390/ijerph15122804

Srygley, J. M., Mirelman, A., Herman, T., Giladi, N.,
& Hausdorff, J. M. (2009). When does walking alter
thinking? Age and task associated findings. *Brain
Research*, *1253*, 92–99.
https://doi.org/10.1016/j.brainres.2008.11.067

Straker, L., Levine, J., & Campbell, A. (2009). The
Effects of Walking and Cycling Computer
Workstations on Keyboard and Mouse Performance.
*Human Factors: The Journal of the Human Factors
and Ergonomics Society*, *51*(6), 831–844.
https://doi.org/10.1177/0018720810362079

Styns, F., van Noorden, L., Moelants, D., & Leman,
M. (2007). Walking on music. *Human Movement*

Science, 26(5), 769–785.
https://doi.org/10.1016/j.humov.2007.07.007

Taylor, A., & Katomeri, M. (2007). Walking reduces cue-elicited cigarette cravings and withdrawal symptoms, and delays ad libitum smoking. *Nicotine & Tobacco Research, 9*(11), 1183–1190.
https://doi.org/10.1080/14622200701648896

Thøgersen-Ntoumani, C., Loughren, E. A., Taylor, I. M., Duda, J. L., & Fox, K. R. (2014). A step in the right direction? Change in mental well-being and self-reported work performance among physically inactive university employees during a walking intervention. *Mental Health and Physical Activity, 7*(2), 89–94.
https://doi.org/10.1016/j.mhpa.2014.06.004

Toomingas, A., Forsman, M., Mathiassen, S. E., Heiden, M., & Nilsson, T. (2012). Variation between seated and standing/walking postures among male and female call centre operators. *BMC Public Health, 12*(1), 0. https://doi.org/10.1186/1471-2458-12-154

Tsetsonis, Natassav., & Hardman, Adrianne. E. (1996). Reduction in postprandial lipemia after

walking: influence of exercise intensity. *Medicine &
Science in Sports & Exercise, 28*(10), 1235–1242.
https://doi.org/10.1097/00005768-199610000-
00005

UK Government. (2020, April 28). *Health matters:
obesity and the food environment.* GOV.UK.
https://www.gov.uk/government/publications/healt
h-matters-obesity-and-the-food-
environment/health-matters-obesity-and-the-food-
environment--
2#:%7E:text=The%20overall%20cost%20of%20obes
ity,%C2%A349.9%20billion%20per%20year.

van Tilburg, W. A. P., & Igou, E. R. (2011). On
boredom: Lack of challenge and meaning as distinct
boredom experiences. *Motivation and Emotion,
36*(2), 181–194. https://doi.org/10.1007/s11031-011-
9234-9

Voss. (2010). Plasticity of brain networks in a
randomized intervention trial of exercise training in
older adults. *Frontiers in Aging Neuroscience,* 0.
https://doi.org/10.3389/fnagi.2010.00032

Waddington, G., Dickson, T., Trathen, S., & Adams, R. (2011). Walking for fitness: is it enough to maintain both heart and bone health? *Australian Journal of Primary Health, 17*(1), 86. https://doi.org/10.1071/py10035

Walking. The creative and mindful space between one step and another | HERMAN BASHIRON MENDOLICCHIO | Walking Art / Walking Aesthetics. (2020). Interartive. https://walkingart.interartive.org/2018/12/hbm-walking

Whitham, J., & Hunt, Y. (2010). The green shoots of good health. *Mental Health Practice, 13*(10), 24–25. https://doi.org/10.7748/mhp2010.07.13.10.24.c7855

Williams, C. L., & Tappen, R. M. (2008). Exercise training for depressed older adults with Alzheimer's disease. *Aging & Mental Health, 12*(1), 72–80. https://doi.org/10.1080/13607860701529932

Williams, P. T. (2013). Walking and Running Produce Similar Reductions in Cause-Specific Disease Mortality in Hypertensives. *Hypertension,*

62(3), 485–491.
https://doi.org/10.1161/hypertensionaha.113.01608

Winchester, J., Dick, M. B., Gillen, D., Reed, B.,
Miller, B., Tinklenberg, J., Mungas, D., Chui, H.,
Galasko, D., Hewett, L., & Cotman, C. W. (2013).
Walking stabilizes cognitive functioning in
Alzheimer's disease (AD) across one year. *Archives of
Gerontology and Geriatrics, 56*(1), 96–103.
https://doi.org/10.1016/j.archger.2012.06.016

Yang, J. F., Stephens, M. J., & Vishram, R. (1998).
Infant stepping: a method to study the sensory
control of human walking. *The Journal of
Physiology, 507*(3), 927–937.
https://doi.org/10.1111/j.1469-7793.1998.927bs.x

Zhou, J., & Hoever, I. J. (2014). Research on
Workplace Creativity: A Review and Redirection.
*Annual Review of Organizational Psychology and
Organizational Behavior, 1*(1), 333–359.
https://doi.org/10.1146/annurev-orgpsych-031413-
091226

At Walking Pace

About the Author

Nyla Naseer lives in Birmingham, United Kingdom. She is a writer and commentator on social change and organisational issues. Her professional life has been complemented by a personal passion for the outdoors.

The dominant themes of Nyla's writing are: the innate need of people to be 'human' in both positive and negative ways, the stories that emerge from the soup of change, and the need to understand how we become influenced by others.

Her non-fiction writing is centred on the tensions between social change and 'human-ness'. Nyla's interest in technology spans legal, economic and technical issues but is most keenly devoted to the impact on individual and social relations. She is a life-long advocate of simplicity, walking and nature and writes about the necessity to revive these elements as part of a human-centred life.

Nyla has a BSc in Management Science, a Master of Science degree in Urban Regeneration and a Master of Law degree. She is also a PGCE qualified trainer, a qualified personal fitness trainer and a certified NLP practitioner.

Away from her writing she can still frequently be seen pounding the paths as a long-distance hiker.

At Walking Pace

www.ingramcontent.com/pod-product-compliance
Lightning Source LLC
Chambersburg PA
CBHW020254030426
42336CB00010B/751